Molecular and Translational Medicine

Series Editors
William B. Coleman
Gregory J. Tsongalis

More information about this series at http://www.springer.com/series/8176

Paula E. North • Tara Sander

Editors

Vascular Tumors and Developmental Malformations

Pathogenic Mechanisms and Molecular Diagnosis

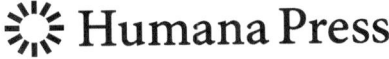 Humana Press

Editors
Paula E. North
Department of Pathology, Division of
  Pediatric Pathology
Medical College of Wisconsin
Milwaukee, WI, USA

Tara Sander
Department of Pathology, Division of
  Pediatric Pathology
Medical College of Wisconsin
Milwaukee, WI, USA

ISSN 2197-7852   ISSN 2197-7860   (electronic)
Molecular and Translational Medicine
ISBN 978-1-4939-3239-9   ISBN 978-1-4939-3240-5   (eBook)
DOI 10.1007/978-1-4939-3240-5

Library of Congress Control Number: 2015956616

Springer New York Heidelberg Dordrecht London

Printed on acid-free paper

Humana Press is a brand of Springer
Springer Science+Business Media LLC New York is part of Springer Science+Business Media
(www.springer.com)

Preface

Vascular anomalies encompass a dizzying array of distinct clinicopathologic entities that can be grouped, roughly, into two general categories: vascular tumors and developmental vascular malformations. The vascular tumors are intrinsically proliferative lesions, at least in some phase of their inception, and include both benign and malignant neoplasms as well as reactive proliferations. The vascular malformations are more static congenital errors in development of the vasculature that may evolve over time under environmental and/or genetic influences. Many of these anomalies, even those officially "benign," can be absolutely devastating for patients over the course of a childhood or a lifetime, also placing great burden on families and frustrating healthcare providers who struggle to provide relief. Current mainstream treatment options are relatively limited, often ineffective, and may be accompanied by significant clinical complications. Surgery and/or interventional radiological approaches are sometimes good solutions, but effective medical intervention would be a much better option for many patients. Design of rational targets for such medical intervention requires understanding of mechanisms of disease. Fortunately, discovery in that regard is escalating.

In this book we bring together a complimentary group of authors representing clinical practice, surgical pathology, molecular diagnostics, and basic science to present different aspects of the puzzle of vascular anomalies. We believe the timing is right, as pieces of this puzzle are now rapidly beginning to fall together. Interest in vascular anomalies is increasing among clinicians and scientists alike, spurred in part by new basic science discoveries as well as by recent beneficial use of "old" drugs like propranolol and rapamycin for new purposes in this field. More and more, basic scientists focused upon vasculogenesis and angiogenesis are attracted by meaningful translational applications in the field of vascular anomalies in addition to other medical fields such as cancer and wound healing. Multidisciplinary centers for the diagnosis, treatment, and study of vascular anomalies have sprung up worldwide. The marvelous new tools we now have for next-generation sequencing and highly sensitive PCR have opened up previously unavailable opportunity for rapid discovery of germline and/or somatic mutations that underlie the development of many vascular anomalies and for development of useful molecular clinical diagnostic tests.

We would like to thank our families and colleagues, of course, for patience and assistance as we and our partnering authors have tried to bring together key elements from an enormous amount of collective information in a rapidly evolving field, still plentiful of collegial controversy to be certain. On that note, we would also like to acknowledge the critical role of the International Society for the Study of Vascular Anomalies (ISSVA) and its global membership in bringing vascular anomalies into the light of international, multidisciplinary scrutiny and consensus for the past three decades. By bringing clinicians, radiologists, pathologists, and basic scientists together to talk and present science regularly, ISSVA has done a great service. Most of all, we would like to thank our patients and their families – they are the real inspiration and driving force behind this most difficult and perplexing of medical fields. Together, we are making progress.

Milwaukee, WI, USA   Paula North
                                                                                Tara Sander

Contents

Contributors

David Bick Pediatrics Department, Medical College of Wisconsin, Milwaukee, WI, USA

Chang Zoon Chun Department of Medicine, Division of Nephrology, Hypertension, & Renal Transplantation, University of Florida, Gainesville, FL, USA

Beth A. Drolet Dermatology Department, Division of Pediatric Dermatology, Medical College of Wisconsin, Milwaukee, WI, USA

Kelly J. Duffy Department of Radiology, Medical College of Wisconsin, Milwaukee, WI, USA

Kristin E. Holland Pediatric Dermatology–Administrative Research Offices, Medical College of Wisconsin, Milwaukee, WI, USA

Michael E. Kelly Pediatrics Department, Division of Pediatric Hematology, Oncology, Bone Marrow Transplantation, Children's Hospital of Wisconsin, Milwaukee, WI, USA

Paula E. North Department of Pathology and Laboratory Medicine, Children's Hospital of Wisconsin, Milwaukee, WI, USA

Department of Pathology, Division of Pediatric Pathology, Medical College of Wisconsin, Milwaukee, WI, USA

Ramani Ramchandran Departments of Pediatrics, and Obstetrics and Gynecology, Neonatology, Medical College of Wisconsin, Inc., Milwaukee, WI, USA

Tara Sander Department of Pathology and Laboratory Medicine, Children's Hospital of Wisconsin, Milwaukee, WI, USA

Department of Pathology, Division of Pediatric Pathology, Medical College of Wisconsin, Milwaukee, WI, USA

Rashmi Sood Department of Pathology, Medical College of Wisconsin, Inc., Milwaukee, WI, USA

Sara Szabo Department of Pathology and Laboratory Medicine, Children's Hospital of Wisconsin, Milwaukee, WI, USA

Department of Pathology, Division of Pediatric Pathology, Medical College of Wisconsin, Milwaukee, WI, USA

Monte S. Willis Pathology & Laboratory Medicine; McAllister Heart Institute, University of North Carolina/UNC Hospitals, Chapel Hill, NC, USA

Chapter 1
Histopathology and Pathogenesis of Vascular Tumors and Malformations

Sara Szabo and Paula E. North

Introduction

Accurate histopathological description combined with knowledgeable clinical and radiological evaluation is an absolute requisite for study and meaningful diagnosis of vascular anomalies, both neoplastic and malformative. Unfortunately, traditional over-generic use of the *hemangioma* has caused inappropriate lumping of entities that we now know are both biologically and clinically dissimilar. Recognizing this problem, the multidisciplinary International Society for the Study of Vascular Anomalies (ISSVA) agreed in 1996 upon the general framework of a biologically based nosologic classification system derived in part from that proposed by Mulliken and Glowacki in which vascular anomalies, based on the presence or absence of endothelial mitotic activity, were divided into tumors and malformations [1]. According to this simplified scheme, the suffix *-angioma* (as in *hemangioma*) should be reserved for benign vascular tumors – whether congenital or acquired, monoclonal or polyclonal – that arise by cellular hyperplasia. On the other hand, the

S. Szabo, MD, PhD • P.E. North, MD, PhD (✉)
Department of Pathology and Laboratory Medicine, Children's Hospital of Wisconsin, 9000 W. Wisconsin Ave, Milwaukee, WI 53226, USA

Department of Pathology, Division of Pediatric Pathology, Medical College of Wisconsin, Milwaukee, WI, USA
e-mail: sszabo@mcw.edu; pnorth@mcw.edu

© Springer Science+Business Media New York 2016
P.E. North, T. Sander (eds.), *Vascular Tumors and Developmental Malformations*, Molecular and Translational Medicine, DOI 10.1007/978-1-4939-3240-5_1

term *malformation* should designate errors in vascular morphogenesis, usually (but not always) clinically evident at birth, that exhibit growth proportional to (+/−) with the patient and little endothelial mitotic activity, e.g., venous malformation.

Refinements in and additions to the new ISSVA-sanctioned classification, most recently updated in 2014 [2], have and will continue to be necessary as lesions that defy classification based on simple criteria are dealt with and as discoveries in vascular biology and genetics continue, but this approach has proved itself in practice internationally to be a useful and rational starting point in a biology-based system for histopathological diagnosis. Accumulated experience has proved that the presence of endothelial mitotic activity alone is not sufficient as a single factor to separate tumors from malformations, since there are secondary effects such as ischemia and turbulence that may stimulate mitotic activity. When combined with correlations with other histological features and clinical behavior, however, consideration of endothelial mitotic activity was a rational starting point that has enlightened our approach to these perplexing lesions.

Although seemingly obvious, this distinction between "angiomas" and malformations represents a significant departure from the traditional diagnostic approach in which the term *hemangioma* was over-applied without regard to etiology or clinical behavior, at best modified by morphological descriptors such as *cavernous* and *capillary*. For instance, even today many experienced pathologists refer to *venous malformations*, which consist of mitotically quiescent collections of developmentally abnormal veins, as *cavernous hemangiomas*. Similarly, developmental abnormalities of lymphatic vessel beds (*lymphatic malformations* by the new scheme) have previously been referred to as *lymphangiomas*, and *arteriovenous malformations* as *arteriovenous hemangiomas*. This poor traditional nosology stems from lack of etiological clarity in the past, but its continued use tends to perpetuate past misconceptions even in the face of new understanding.

It is important to reemphasize that precise histopathological diagnosis of the various types of vascular anomalies does in fact play an important role in clinical management of patients. This is not just an exercise in pigeonholing. Among the vascular malformations, for instance, some respond well to sclerotherapy, while others do not; some are likely to recur with renewed strength if not completely excised, and others are not; some are associated with progressive soft tissue and bony overgrowth, and others are not; and so on. Likewise, among the so-called capillary hemangiomas, some entities will spontaneously regress, whereas others will not; some are likely to cause coagulopathy, while others are not; some skin lesions are almost certainly associated with gastrointestinal or other underlying visceral lesions, and others are not; some respond to steroids, and others do not. Despite the fact that "capillary hemangiomas" share composition by capillary-sized vessels, they are distinguishable not only in histological detail, but by their molecular expression patterns. Thus, beyond the need to separate *hemangioma* and other tumors from *malformation*, it is evident that the term *hemangioma*, even when modified by *capillary*, does not function well as a stand-alone diagnosis. Instead, pathologists and clinicians alike must modify it, whenever possible, using descriptors that clearly indicate the specific clinicopathological entity intended (i.e., infantile hemangioma, non-involuting congenital hemangioma, spindle cell hemangioma, etc.).

This chapter provides an overview of the current clinical, histological, and immunophenotypical features that distinguish the major types of vascular tumors and malformations presenting in infancy and childhood and summarizes the diagnostic histopathological criteria and nomenclature currently applied to these lesions in most major vascular anomalies centers around the world. A general discussion of pathogenesis is also included for most entities, providing correlation between clinical, epidemiological, histo-immunophenotypic, and, for many, genetic features. Molecular diagnostic considerations and clinical management approaches are presented in more depth in Chaps. 4 and 5, respectively. The histopathological classification presented here is congruent with the latest ISSVA consensus statement [2]. Discussion opens with the vascular tumors and tumorlike lesions and ends with the vascular malformations.

Vascular Tumors and Tumorlike Lesions

Classically, vascular tumors, as originally defined by ISSVA, arise by cellular hyperplasia and show disproportionate growth compared to that of the child. This is in contrast to vascular malformations, which develop in utero as errors in vascular morphogenesis and typically grow in proportion to the child. Specialists in the field recognize, however, that this is not a clean division. For instance, some vascular "tumors" per the latest ISSVA classification [2] are congenitally fully formed and typically do not show disproportionate postnatal growth – these are the congenital nonprogressive hemangiomas subcategorized by the anacronyms *RICH, NICH, and PICH*. Until we better understand the pathogenesis of these latter lesions, they are perhaps best discussed provisionally as "tumorlike" lesions, as done in this section. It should be noted that many clinically important vascular tumorlike lesions are not included at all in the WHO classification of soft tissue tumors, including the congenital nonprogressive hemangiomas. Histopathological features of the major categories of vascular tumors and tumorlike lesions are discussed below, accompanied by brief clinical and pathogenic information for orientation. Discussion begins with infantile hemangioma (IH), the most common type of vascular tumor and, in fact, the most common tumor of infancy. Several other histologically and clinically distinct types of vascular tumors and tumorlike lesions that typically present in early childhood or during gestation are then addressed. Some of these are life-threatening and all are important to diagnose precisely so that appropriate therapies can be applied. Those with established infectious etiology, including Kaposi's sarcoma, bacillary angiomatosis, and verruga peruana, and those commonly thought to be reactive vascular proliferations, including so-called pyogenic granuloma, glomeruloid hemangioma, microvenular hemangioma, and reactive angioendotheliomatosis, are omitted.

Benign Vascular Tumors and Tumorlike Lesions

Infantile Hemangioma (IH)

Clinical Features

Infantile hemangioma (IH) is the most common tumor of infancy, affecting approximately 4 % of children, with a threefold female-to-male ratio. Commonly used synonyms include *juvenile hemangioma* and *cellular hemangioma of infancy*. Hemangiomas of this type display a remarkably predictable natural course: they present shortly after birth with rapid growth in the first year of life, followed by slow spontaneous involution over a period of years. Fair-skinned individuals are at increased risk, although all races are affected, as are low birth weight infants [3, 4].

Although all IH spontaneously involute to a variable degree and with variable speed over a period of years, significant cosmetic or functional sequelae are not uncommon [5, 6]. Complications during the proliferative phase may include cutaneous ulceration, bleeding, infection, airway compromise, jaw malalignment, and, rarely, congestive heart failure [6]. Periorbital lesions blocking the visual axis may cause amblyopia. Infants with diffuse hepatic involvement by IH may develop severe hypothyroidism due to tumoral expression of type 3 iodothyronine deiodinase [7].

IH display a number of intriguing anatomical predilections and patterns of tissue involvement which may hold pathogenic clues. Approximately 60 % occur on the head and neck, although they also occur on the trunk, extremities, genitals, and in various viscera including notably the liver, the intestine, and less often the lung. Skin and subcutis appear to be most commonly affected, even considering the more obvious presentation, whereas deep skeletal muscle is spared. True IH do not appear to arise within brain parenchyma, but can involve the tissues investing leptomeningeal vessels and thus be intracranial. Most present as solitary cutaneous and/or subcutaneous lesions, but a significant percentage of patients (about 15 %) have multiple skin lesions, in rare cases accompanied by multiple visceral hemangiomas (usually hepatic), intuitively suggesting "dissemination." Although most IH of skin and subcutis appear as focal masses, others show a more plaque-like pattern with a distinctly segmental distribution [8]. Segmental facial IH may occur in association with one or more of the following abnormalities: posterior fossa brain malformations, arterial cerebrovascular anomalies, cardiovascular anomalies, and eye anomalies, described by the acronym PHACE syndrome, or PHACES syndrome when accompanied by sternal defects and/or supraumbilical raphe [9]. The etiology of this association is not understood, but it is possible that the IH may be a secondary occurrence in a developmentally altered segment. PHACE patients with cerebrovascular anomalies are at risk for progressive vasculopathy leading to stenotic and occlusive changes and rare risk of ischemic stroke [10]. Analogously, lower body segmental cutaneous IH have been described in association with regional congenital analogies by the suggested acronym of LUMBAR syndrome [11].

As a treatment choice, innocuous lesions are generally left alone to involute spontaneously. To prevent or mitigate clinically significant complications, surgical excision and medical treatment options are considered. Since the initial report in 2008 of its use for medical treatment of IH, propranolol has been rapidly adopted for this purpose, although not without significant potential side effects [12, 13]. Other medical therapies include corticosteroids (topical, intralesional, and systemic), pulsed-dye laser, and imiquimod (topical, for superficial lesions). The use of recombinant interferon-alpha is restricted to life-threatening lesions due to the risk of rare but irreversible spastic diplegia. Large involuted tumors may be excised for cosmetic reasons. For some clinically problematic proliferative phase IH, for instance, those blocking the visual axis, surgical excision may be preferable to medical therapy [14].

Histology

Proliferative phase IH [15, 16] consist of cellular masses of capillaries, with small rounded lumina, lined by plump endothelial cells that are surrounded by pericytes (Fig. 1.1); both cell types show occasional mitoses. Interspersed are pericapillary immature dendritic-type cells. The basement membrane becomes multi-laminated over time. The proliferating capillaries are arranged in lobules, which are separated by delicate fibrous septa or normal intervening tissue (Fig. 1.2). Lesional capillaries intermingle nondestructively with normal structures (superficial skeletal muscle fibers, adipocytes, skin adnexa, peripheral nerves, and salivary glands). As a result of high blood flow, draining veins become enlarged, with thickened asymmetrical walls. IH do not show intravascular thrombosis, hemosiderin deposition, or necrosis – unless secondary to ulceration or presurgical embolization.

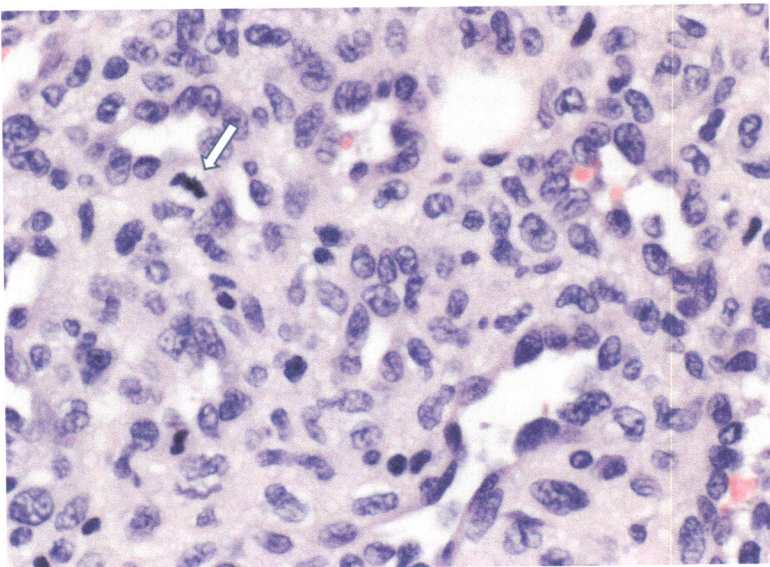

Fig. 1.1 Infantile hemangioma, proliferative phase. Endothelial cells and pericytes together form plump, tightly packed capillaries. Note the mitotic figure (*arrow*)

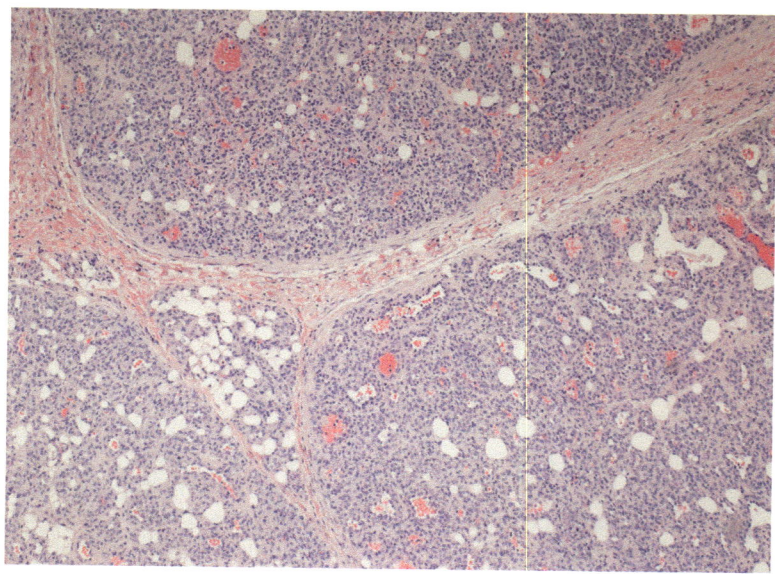

Fig. 1.2 Infantile hemangioma, proliferative phase, characteristic lobularity. Capillary lobules in this cutaneous example are separated by normal intervening dermal stroma

In the involuting phase, lesional capillaries gradually disappear, basement membranes thicken and show embedded apoptotic dust, and pericapillary mast cells increase in number (Fig. 1.3). As previously stated, thrombosis and inflammation are not significant features. In the late involuting phase, near end stage, lobules are replaced by loose fibrous or fibrofatty stroma, with only few residual vessels, which remarkably preserve their immunophenotype. "Ghost" vessels show thickened multilayered rinds of basement membrane material, with apoptotic debris and little or no intact cellular lining (Fig. 1.4). Previously ulcerated lesions show epidermal atrophy and fibrous scarring. Large arteries and draining veins do not completely regress. This phenomenon, paired with diminution of mitotic activity, may lead to mistaken diagnosis of the lesion as a vascular malformation (Fig. 1.5). This misinterpretation can usually be avoided by consideration of clinical history and overall histological appearance.

Immunohistochemical studies of IH (Fig. 1.6) have revealed a unique and complex endothelial phenotype for IH that is shared only by placental capillaries, including strong expression of GLUT1, Lewis Y antigen, Fc gamma receptor II, CD15, CCR6, IDO, and IGF2 [15, 17–19]. The basement membrane of IH capillaries is strongly enriched in merosin, also characteristic of placental capillaries [18]. This is a committed endothelial phenotype for which most of these placenta-associated markers persist throughout the natural course of IH. As a result, GLUT1 immunohistochemistry in particular has become extremely useful for diagnostic confirmation of IH and is widely considered the international gold standard for that purpose. One must exercise caution to differentiate the strongly GLUT1-positive circulating

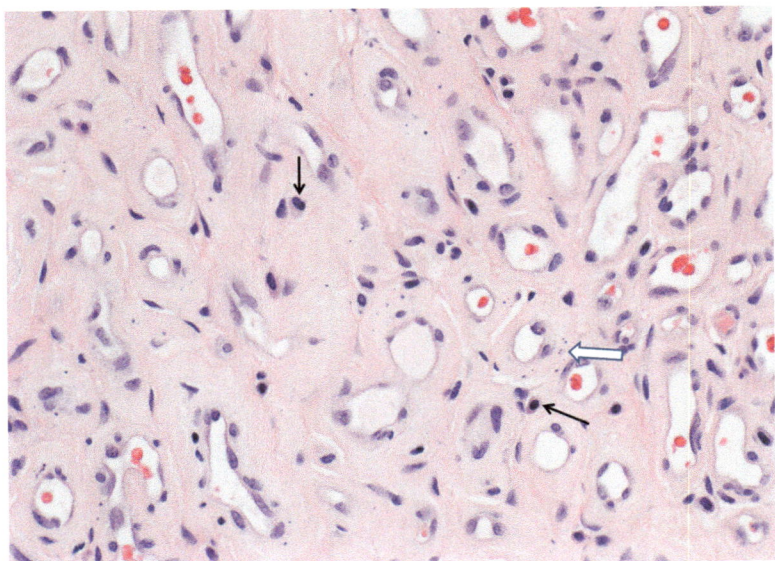

Fig. 1.3 Infantile hemangioma, actively involuting phase. Note the thickened capillary basement membranes containing apoptotic debris (*thick arrow*). Pericapillary mast cells are numerous (*thin arrows*)

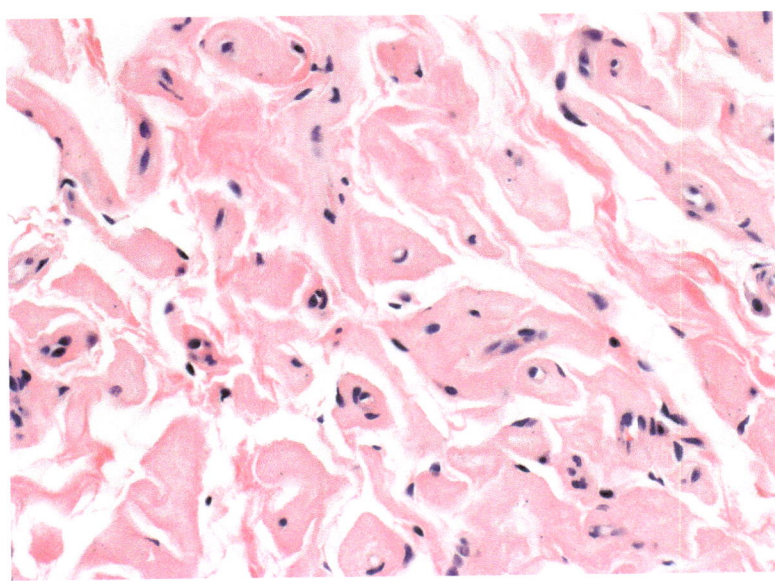

Fig. 1.4 Infantile hemangioma, late involuting stage. Basement membranes of residual capillaries are thick and hyalinized

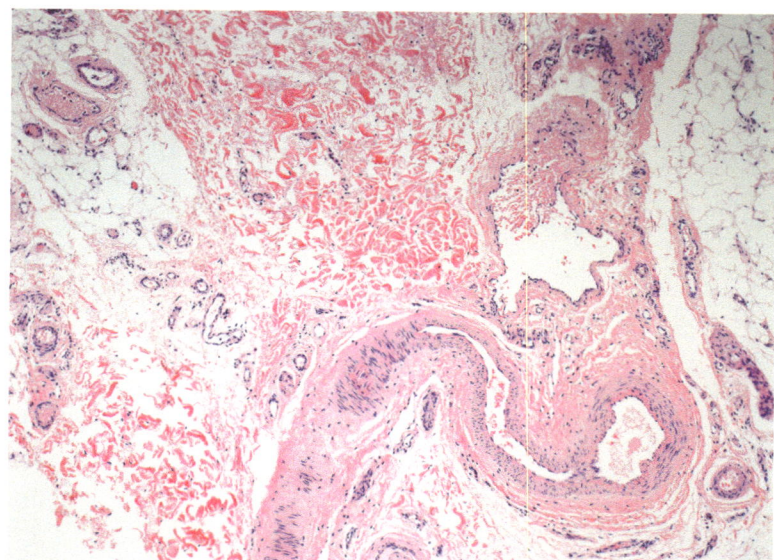

Fig. 1.5 Infantile hemangioma, end stage. Residual feeding and draining vessels persist after capillaries drop out, lending appearance similar to that of a vascular malformation

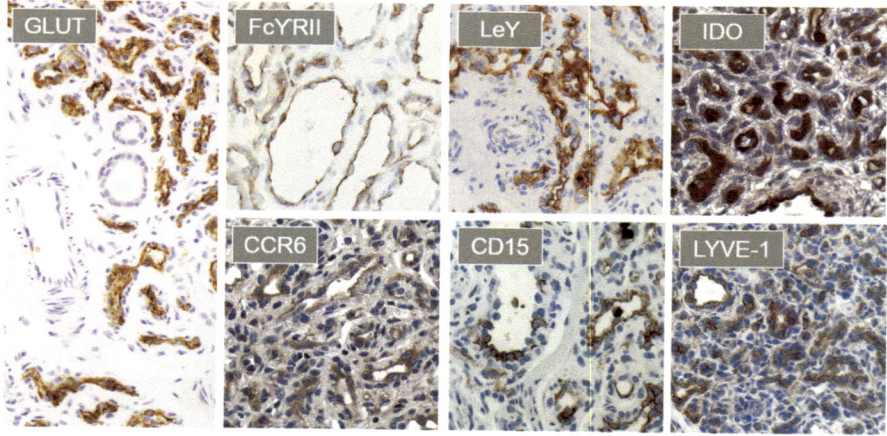

Fig. 1.6 Infantile hemangioma, unique capillary immunophenotype shared by placental capillaries

erythrocytes, or their degeneration products, from endothelial positivity (or the lack of it.) Lesional capillaries of IH are also positive for "normal" endothelial markers of the blood vasculature (including CD31, CD34, vWf, *Ulex europaeus* lectin I, Fli-1, ERG, and VE-cadherin).

Pathogenesis

Rare families with frequent IH have shown linkage to chromosome 5q31-33, suggesting potential influential mutations [20, 21]. Nevertheless, IH are very common and the vast majority of IH are sporadic, casting doubt that IH is a genetic disease. IH are notably more common in low birth weight infants and twins, but lack of concordance in twin studies also argues against a strongly predisposing inherited component [22]. Although all races are affected by IH, being Caucasian, female, or fair-haired appears to lower the threshold for hemangiogenesis, mechanisms for which are completely unknown.

Independent of consideration of potential genetic determinants or modulators of IH, which seem likely to be weak at best, the unusual molecular signature that is curiously shared only by IH capillaries and the fetal capillaries of placental villi has generated much etiological discussion. Current evidence favors the hypothesis that IH arises from multipotent vascular precursor cells, which quite possibly may originate from in the placenta [15, 17, 18, 23–28]. It is also intriguing that the phenotype of placental and IH endothelial cells, exemplified by CD31, CD34, GLUT1, Lewis Y antigen, IDO, CD15, and FcγRII co-expression, shows great overlap with that of early hematopoietic and vasculogenic cells and in part with mature cells of the myelo-monocytic lineage [15, 18]. These shared patterns of expression emphasize the close ontological relation between hematopoietic and vascular development that begins in the yolk sac and continues into the adult bone marrow and support the supposition that the endothelial cells of both IH and placenta are "arrested," if you will (presumably by evolutionary plan in the case of placenta), in a specialized, intermediate state of vascular/hematopoietic differentiation that must have selective advantage in the case of the placenta [18, 25, 29]. A recent study by Jinnin et al. reported low VEGFR1 expression in cultured endothelial cells from IH, compared to various controls, with resultant activation of VEGRF2 and its downstream targets [30]. This may have significant therapeutic implications, as yet uninvestigated. It is probable that extraneous systemic factors impact the behavior of IH; a recent study reported regrowth of IH in late childhood in two patients on exogenous growth hormone therapy [31].

Congenital Nonprogressive Hemangiomas: Rapidly Involuting Congenital Hemangioma (RICH) and Non-involuting Congenital Hemangioma (NICH)

Clinical Features

Congenital nonprogressive hemangiomas are congenital lesions that, unlike IH, are fully formed at birth and then typically follow either static clinical course (non-involuting congenital hemangioma/*NICH*) or a very rapidly regressive course in 3–5 months due to infarction (rapidly involuting congenital hemangioma/*RICH*) [32–34]. Only exceptional examples show limited progressive clinical growth, and they occur with equal sex predilection (as for vascular malformations). There is considerable histological overlap between the *NICH* and *RICH* clinical subtypes; current opinion favors that they are biologically synonymous entities that vary primarily in propensity for infarction and thus regression. In fact, some lesions of this type only partially regress and have been dubbed partially involuting congenital hemangioma *(PICH)* [35]. Most lesions are cutaneous and/or subcutaneous. Visceral lesions are typically solitary and centrally necrotic lesions, most in the liver, occasionally in the brain. Reportedly multifocal visceral lesions have been poorly documented histologically. MRI reveals well-circumscribed masses with large flow voids reminiscent of arteriovenous malformation (AVM). Regressing lesions show central necrosis, often with superimposed calcification. Complications are impacted by location and size and include hemorrhage, scarring, atrophy, and for large lesions high-output heart failure [36]. During central infarction and lesional regression, large RICH may be complicated by transient mild-to-moderate thrombocytopenia and consumptive coagulopathy.

Histology

Histological features of RICH and NICH vary along a spectrum of change, dependent largely upon the degree of infarction, with PICH as an intermediate state. To emphasize this spectrum, it is good practice for pathologists to provide a diagnosis of *congenital nonprogressive hemangioma*, modified as either the *rapidly involuting (RICH) or non-involuting (NICH) clinical variant*. The term *PICH* is used less often.

Whether rapidly involuting or non-involuting, congenital nonprogressive hemangiomas are typically comprised of variably circumscribed capillary lobules separated by abnormally dense fibrous tissue, with frequent atrophy and loss of dermal adnexal appendages in involved and overlying skin (Fig. 1.7). This contrasts with IH, where tumor lobules are separated by normal-appearing tissue elements (Fig. 1.2). Endothelial cells and pericytes within the capillary lobules can be moderately plump, focally resembling those of proliferative phase IH but lacking increased endothelial mitotic activity and multi-lamination of basement membranes (Fig. 1.8). The lobules often show stellate thin-walled, centrilobular, draining vessels and may be peripherally or globally sclerotic (Fig. 1.9). Other common features are thrombosis, foci of hemosiderin deposition and/or extramedullary hematopoiesis, thrombosis, and calcification. There is typically a prominent interlobular vascular network of venous arterial and often lymphatic channels that may be more prominent than the more cellular capillary lobules in some cases, which must be differentiated from vascular malformation (Fig. 1.10). Grossly evident areas of central depression and scarring in regressing lesions appear to correlate with a central core that contains large central draining channels and few capillary lobules. Features more commonly seen in NICH than RICH are hobnailed endothelium, large and loosely defined capillary lobules, and arteriovenous fistulas [32, 34]. The residual lesion of RICH of peripheral soft tissues is characterized by cutaneous and subcutaneous collapse with variable loss of dermal and adipose tissue that may extend down to the level of the muscle fascia. In both RICH and NICH, the lesional endothelial cells are negative for GLUT1 and the other distinctive markers of IH (Fig. 1.11) [32].

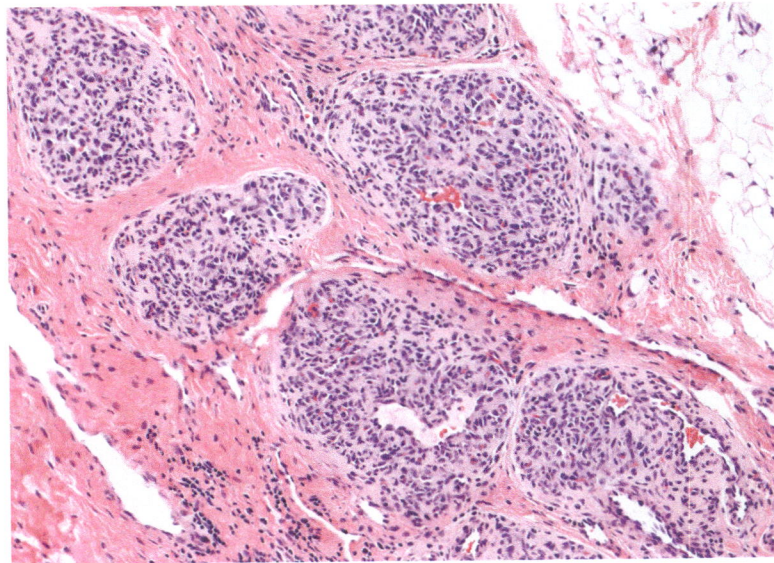

Fig. 1.7 Congenital nonprogressive hemangioma. Capillary lobules are separated by fibrotic stroma

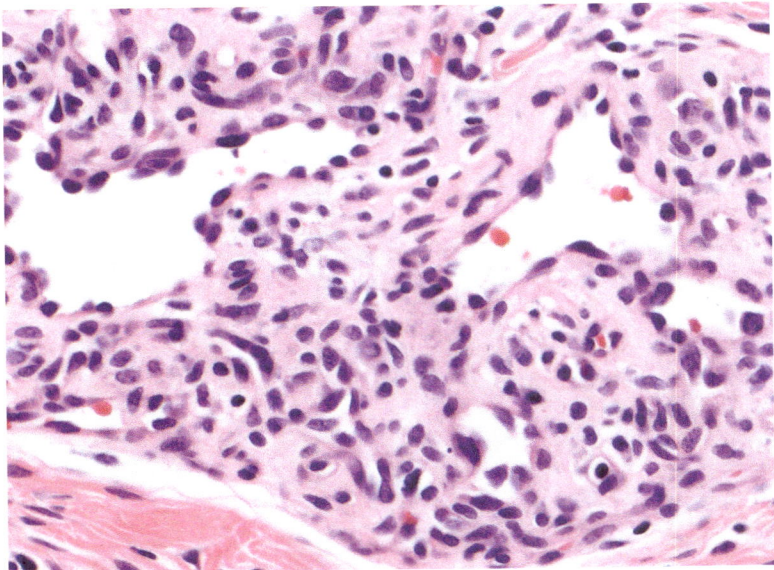

Fig. 1.8 Congenital nonprogressive hemangioma, high magnification. Endothelial cells may be plump, but generally lack mitotic activity

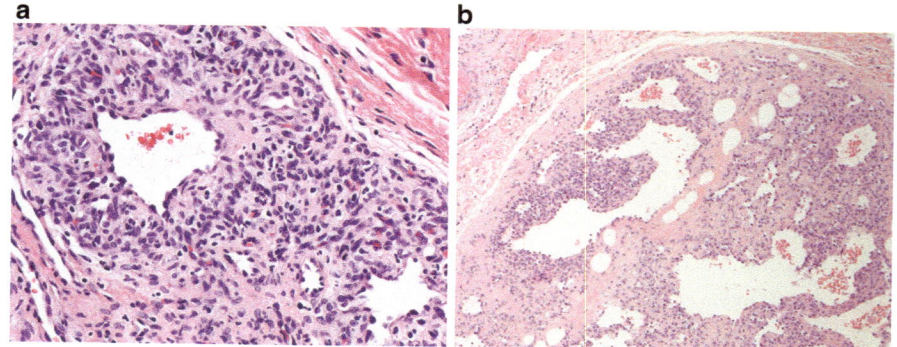

Fig. 1.9 Congenital nonprogressive hemangioma, lobules. (**a**) Many have stellate draining vessels. (**b**) Lobular sclerosis is common

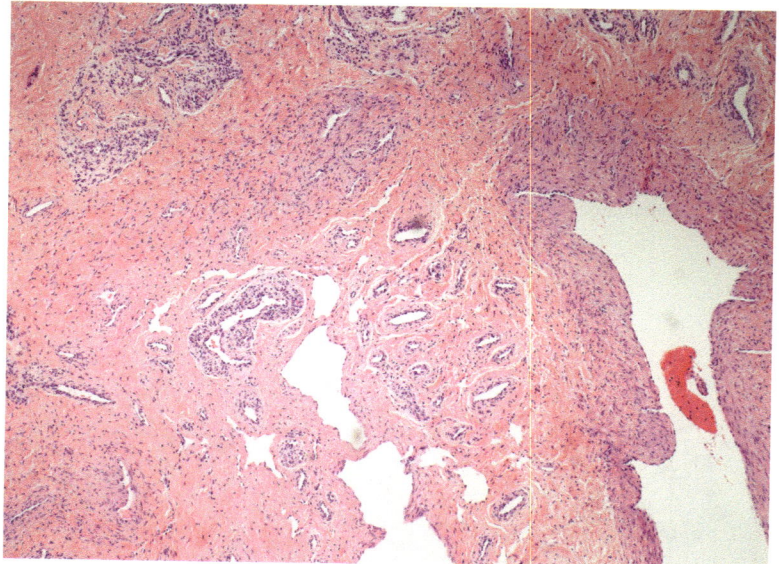

Fig. 1.10 Congenital nonprogressive hemangioma, prominent septal vasculature

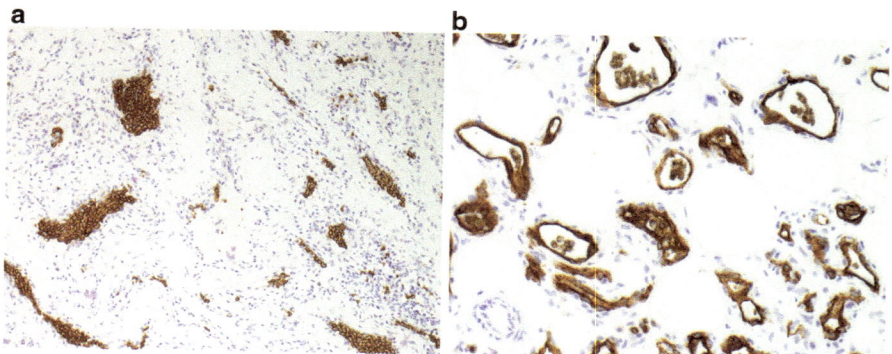

Fig. 1.11 Congenital nonprogressive hemangioma (**a**) vs infantile hemangioma (**b**), GLUT1 immunoreaction

Pathogenesis

The pathogenesis of congenital nonprogressive hemangiomas is unknown, other than the contribution of infarction to regression, but clearly this family of lesions (*RICH, NICH, and PICH*) is biologically unrelated to classical IH, based upon strongly differing histological features and immunophenotype as well as clinical presentation and behavior. The histology of the capillary lobules of these lesions bears some resemblance to that of acquired so-called pyogenic granulomas that are sometimes associated with history of trauma. This suggests the possibility of focal intrauterine vascular accident or tissue injury that spawns a local reparative vascular process in utero. Basically, we don't know. Currently, there is no evidence for, or strong suspicion of, a genetic determinate.

Hepatic Hemangiomas

Clinical Features

Recent experience supports division of benign hemangiomas involving the liver into two major clinicopathological categories, the first being solitary (i.e., "focal") *congenital hepatic hemangioma*, which is analogous to *RICH* in other locations, and the second being *multifocal hepatic infantile hemangioma* (IH), which is equivalent to GLUT1-positive *IH* in other locations [15, 37–39]. In some patients with hepatic IH, multifocal lesions so diffusely involve the liver that they become confluent and present a number of complications not typically seen in cases with less tumoral burden. It has thus been suggested that hepatic hemangiomas include a third category, that of *diffuse hepatic hemangioma* [40].

Hepatic RICH are fully developed intrauterine and are often detected by prenatal ultrasound. They present at birth as a large solitary abdominal mass, not uncommonly complicated by congestive heart failure, anemia, and mild coagulopathy. Magnetic resonance imaging with T2 weighting shows a hyperintense heterogeneous mass with central necrosis and calcification. Imaging is helpful to clinically differentiate these lesions from neonatal tumors, such as hepatoblastoma. If clinical and imaging findings are atypical, biopsy, usually percutaneous, is indicated. Accelerated regression is generally complete in about 1 year, although some residuum or focus of scarring may persist. As such, the treatment of choice for most patients is observation and supportive care for complications as needed. In some cases, other treatment modalities applied with close interdisciplinary collaboration, including pharmacotherapy, hepatic vascular shunt embolization, and resection, may be required [40].

Multifocal hepatic IH range from few small (incidentally discovered) lesions to numerous lesions scattered about the liver causing recognizable hepatomegaly. These may remain clinically occult or may present in the neonatal period with hepatomegaly and cardiopulmonary distress, often with coexistent hemangiomas in the skin and, more rarely, additional viscera. Like cutaneous and subcutaneous forms of this entity, hepatic IH are characterized by early postnatal growth and spontaneous slow involution. Patients with massive, confluent involvement of the liver by IH (i.e., *diffuse hepatic IH*) are subject to potential abdominal compartment syndrome during the proliferative phase and will almost certainly develop clinically significant hypothyroidism due to high tumoral expression of type 3 iodothryonine deiodinase [40, 41]. Since undetected hypothyroidism can decrease cardiac contractility and result in permanent neurologic damage, it is essential that thyroid screening be performed early in these patients, with aggressive initiation of thyroid replacement therapy [40].

Histology

Grossly, hepatic RICH are large, spherical, well-defined hemorrhagic masses with central necrosis and calcification. Microscopic examination reveals a large central area of infarction and hemorrhage surrounded by more cellular zones of capillaries which are encased in fibrous stroma also entrapping bile ducts (Fig. 1.12). Thrombosis and calcification are common, and extramedullary hematopoiesis is usually prominent. Lesional endothelial cells of hepatic RICH are negative for GLUT1 and other distinctive markers of IH.

The histology of *multifocal hepatic infantile hemangioma (IH)* is rarely if ever seen by pathologists past the proliferative phase and is similar to that of proliferative phase IH in skin and subcutis, other than differing tissue elements and background stroma. Cellular but unencapsulated collections of small capillaries with moderately

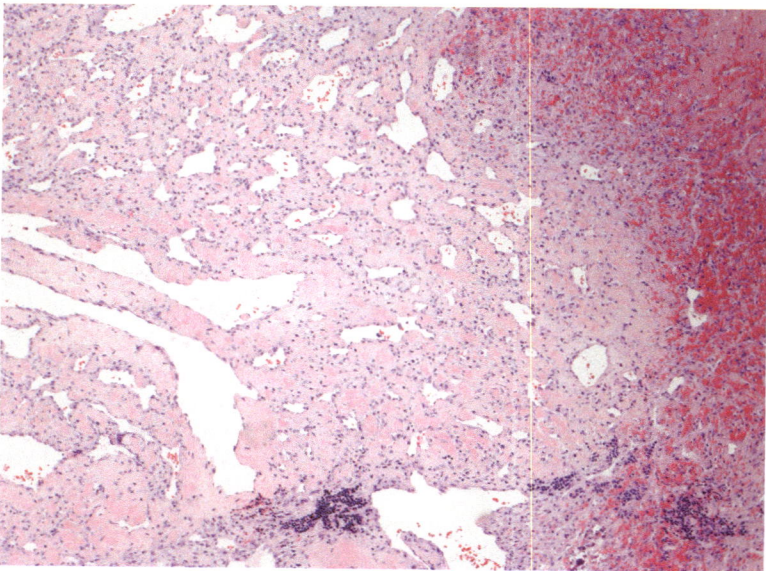

Fig. 1.12 Hepatic RICH-type solitary congenital hemangioma. Note the large area of central infarction and hemorrhage (*right*), rimmed by a more cellular zone with capillaries and scattered small bile ducts trapped in fibrotic stroma

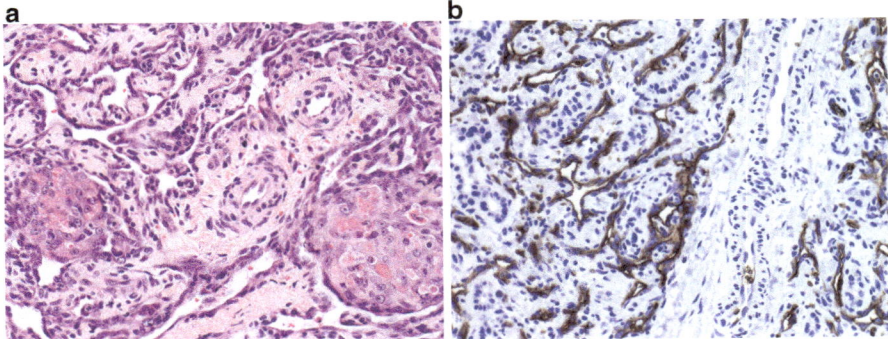

Fig. 1.13 Hepatic infantile hemangioma. (**a**) Well-circumscribed nests of plump capillaries are arranged in a delicate fibrous stroma containing intermingled hepatocytes and small bile ducts. (**b**) As in cutaneous IH, lesional endothelial cells are strongly positive for GLUT1

plump endothelial cells and pericytes are arranged within a delicate fibrous stroma sometimes containing entrapped bile ducts and/or hepatocytes (Fig. 1.13a). In patients with clinically evident hepatomegaly, lesions are multiple and scattered throughout the hepatic parenchyma. Those discovered incidentally, for instance, at autopsy for other causes of death, may be tiny and easily missed upon microscopic examination. Lesional endothelial cells of hepatic IH immunoreact positively for GLUT1 and other markers diagnostic of cutaneous IH (Fig. 1.13b).

Hobnail Hemangioma (Newly Termed Targetoid Hemosiderotic Lymphatic Malformation)

Clinical Features

Hobnail hemangioma, originally described by Santa Cruz and Aronberg in 1988 using the term *targetoid hemosiderotic hemangioma*, is an uncommon, congenital or acquired, benign biphasic cutaneous lesion that typically presents as a red-blue or brown papule, sometimes surrounded by a pale ring and ecchymotic halo, in children and young to middle-aged adults. Most occur on the extremities, but examples on the back, buttock and hip, chest wall, and other sites have been reported. Acquired lesions often have a history of preceding trauma [42]. Excised lesions do not recur.

Histology

Lesions are composed of a superficial dermal compliment of thin-walled vessels with focally hobnailed endothelial cells, merging with a deeper dermal component of smaller slit-like vessels (Fig. 1.14a). Lining endothelial cells are strongly positive for podoplanin and negative or weakly positive for CD34, consistent with pure lymphatic derivation (Fig. 1.14b).

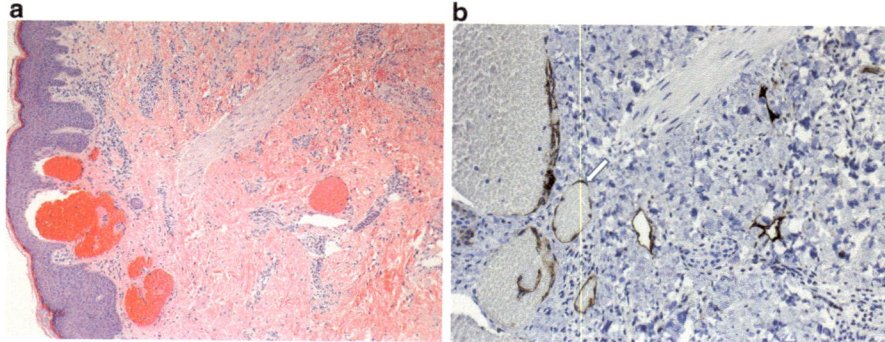

Fig. 1.14 The so-called hobnail hemangioma, now considered a type of lymphatic malformation. (**a**) H&E-stained sections reveal dilated thin-walled vessels with slightly hobnailed endothelium in the superficial dermis, becoming smaller and more angular in the deeper dermis. (**b**) Endothelial cells are strongly positive for podoplanin (*arrow*), consistent with lymphatic differentiation. Mitoses are absent. Hemosiderin deposits are sometimes present in the peripheral dermal stroma (not seen here), imparting a "targetoid hemosiderotic" clinical appearance

Extravasated erythrocytes and hemosiderin deposits are common. Though occasional delicate intraluminal papillary fronds may be seen, the complex endothelial tufts of Dabska-type hemangioendothelioma (see below) are lacking.

Pathogenesis

The lymphatic nature of the lining endothelial cells has been consistently commented upon based on a number of criteria, leading to suggestion that these lesions are in fact "lymphangiomas" [43, 44]. Congruent with ISSVA-sanctioned restriction of the suffix "angioma" to vascular tumors, Dhaybe et al., upon further demonstrating that endothelial cells of hobnail hemangioma are generally negative for Wilms' tumor-1 and demonstrate a low Ki-67 proliferation index, recently suggested that the term *targetoid hemosiderotic lymphatic malformation* be applied to this entity [42]. The presence of microshunts between adjacent lesional lymphatic vessels and small blood vessels may explain observation of erythrocytes within and around the lymphatic vessels of so-called hobnail hemangioma as well as the characteristic stromal hemosiderin deposits [44].

Epithelioid Hemangioma

Clinical Features

Originally termed *angiolymphoid hyperplasia with eosinophilia* when described by Wells and Whimster in 1969 and then later as *histiocytoid hemangioma*, these potentially reactive lesions present as slowly growing angiomatous nodules or plaques, often multiple or grouped, on the head and neck, especially around the ears. Most are dermal and/or subcutaneous, but some occur in deeper tissues, especially the bone [45, 46]. The superficial lesions may be pruritic, painful, and/or pulsatile. Regional lymph node enlargement and peripheral eosinophilia have been reported in some patients. Many cases are associated with arteriovenous shunts, some with history of trauma [45]. Lesions often recur after surgical, laser, or radiation therapy; rare spontaneous regression also has been reported.

Histology

Epithelioid hemangiomas are histologically characterized by usually dermal and subcutaneous, well-circumscribed proliferations of capillary-sized vessels around larger central vessels, with a variably dense lympho-histiocytic and eosinophilic infiltrate (Fig. 1.15). Other commonly observed components are plasma cells and nodular lymphoid aggregates with or without germinal centers. Fibrosis may outweigh the inflammation in older lesions. Many of the capillaries and some larger vessels are lined by enlarged endothelial cells with abundant eosinophilic or amphophilic cytoplasm that protrude into the lumen, imparting a cobblestone appearance and explaining the use of descriptors "epithelioid" and, previously, "histiocytoid." In many specimens, mural damage in a medium to large artery, as evidenced by myxoid degeneration, inflammatory infiltration, or rupture, is present [47]. Pathologists must take care to distinguish epithelioid hemangiomas from potential malignant lookalikes – epithelioid hemangioendothelioma and epithelioid angiosarcoma – especially in the bone [46].

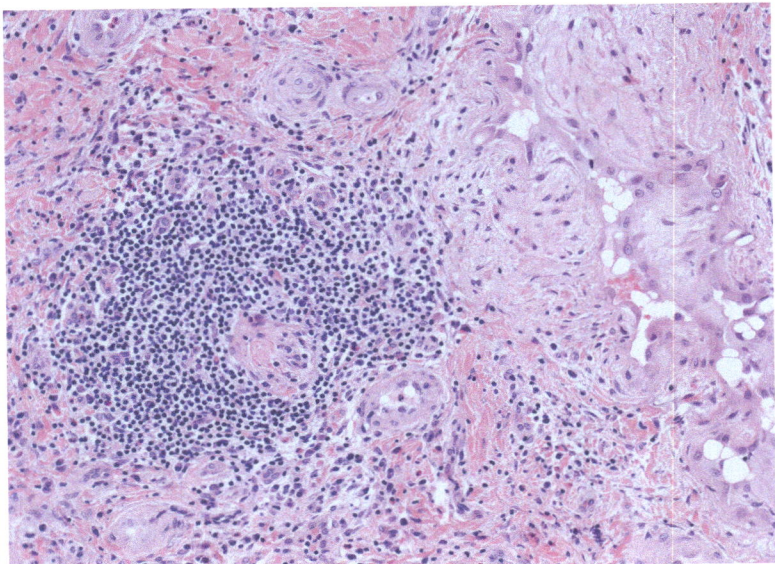

Fig. 1.15 Epithelioid hemangioma

Pathogenesis

Epithelioid hemangioma is classified as a benign vascular tumor by both the WHO and ISSVA [2, 48]. However, several features of these lesions suggest, at a minimum, significant contribution of reactive, as opposed to neoplastic, mechanisms to its pathogenesis. Certainly, the frequent presence of mural damage or rupture in intralesional large vessels has suggested a role of trauma or arteriovenous shunting in its pathogenesis [45]. Similarly, it is of note that lesions interpreted as epithelioid hemangioma have not uncommonly been reported in association with preexisting arteriovenous fistulas and malformations. Perhaps also relevant is the fact that all ages and ethnicities are affected. It is possible that "epithelioid hemangioma" is a heterogeneous group of histologically overlapping disorders, some neoplastic and others reactive to AV-shunting. That is an uncertainty we must live with for the moment. TIE2 (TEK) mutations have been reported in rare cases of epithelioid hemangioma, but that finding has not been corroborated by other studies [49].

Spindle Cell Hemangioma

Clinical Features

Spindle cell hemangioma (SCH) is an acquired lesion developing in children and adults with equal sex distribution that was originally interpreted as a low-grade angiosarcoma and accordingly termed *spindle cell hemangioendothelioma* [50]. Reevaluation over the years lead Perkins and Weiss to rename this lesion *spindle cell hemangioma* in recognition of its benign histological features and lack of metastatic potential [51]. Most present as solitary, firm, red-brown or blue nodular lesions in the skin and subcutis, usually of the distal upper or lower extremity, with growth of the initial lesion and slow development of multifocal lesions in the same general area. They may be asymptomatic or painful. Roughly 60 % recur following excision [51].

Histology

Lesions consist of well-circumscribed nodules characterized by two elements: thin-walled cavernous vascular spaces (veins) containing organizing thrombi and more cellular areas with spindle cells and occasional aggregates of vacuolated epithelioid cells. In some cases, the cellular proliferations of spindled and epithelioid cells are entirely intravascular [51], and about 50 % of cases of SCC have an intravascular component [52]. The epithelioid cells, as well as the flattened cells lining the cavernous vessels, immunoreact for endothelial markers [53], whereas the spindled cells have pericytic and fibroblastic features [53–55].

Pathogenesis

SCH is listed as a benign vascular tumor in the ISSVA classification [2]. Lesions of this histology have been reported in association with a number of types of vascular anomalies (malformations) as well as varicose veins, but are overrepresented in Klippel–Trenaunay syndrome and particularly in Maffucci syndrome [53, 56]. It has widely been considered to be nonneoplastic, possibly a venous malformation dominated by effects of thrombosis organization and irregular vascular collapse. This theory is supported by the associations of SCH with Maffucci and Klippel–Trenaunay syndromes, both of these syndromes also characterized by the presence of venous malformations. Very recently, Amyere et al. reported frequent somatic alterations in 2p22.3, 2q24.3, and 14q11.2 in patients with Maffucci syndrome that may play a role in causing enchondroma and SCH in these patients [56]. Somatic mutations in IDH1 and, more rarely, IDH2 were also recently found in tumoral tissue (including SCH and enchondromas) from 10 of 13 (77 %) of patient's with Maffucci syndrome [57]. Since heterozygous hotshot mutations in IDH1/2 are frequently observed in several types of tumors and cause epigenetic modifications – and these can cause altered pathophysiologic expression of genes – IDH1/2 mutations could potentially affect the development of SCH as well as cartilaginous tumors in Maffucci patients [56, 58].

Vascular Tumors Associated with Selective Thrombocytopenia

Kaposiform Hemangioendothelioma (KHE) and Tufted Angioma (TA)

Clinical Features

The Kasabach–Merritt phenomenon (KMP) was originally defined in 1940 as life-threatening thrombocytopenic purpura occurring in the setting of an enlarging "hemangioma," decades before we recognized the many distinct categories of vascular anomalies that previously were lumped under the term "hemangioma." KMP is characterized by profound sustained thrombocytopenia, sometimes compounded by microangiopathic hemolytic anemia and secondary consumption of fibrinogen and coagulation factors. It differs from the chronic consumptive coagulopathy that can complicate large lymphatic or venous malformations in which platelet counts are normal or only slightly decreased, but fibrinogen and clotting factor levels are low. We now realize that KMP is not caused by the very common IH, even if very large, but instead is a complication of two, possibly synonymous vascular tumors that histologically overlap: *tufted angioma* (TA) and *kaposiform hemangioendothelioma* (KHE) [59, 60]. Many consider KHE and TA to be variants of the same clinicopathological entity, with the term TA arising from the dermatology literature to describe superficial, often less aggressive examples of KHE. Unlike IH, which shows strong female predilection, KHE and TA are equally prevalent in males and females.

Preferred locations of the KHE/TA spectrum include the skin and subcutis, deep soft tissues, bone, and spleen. Rare cases of KMP have been reported in patients with congenital fibrosarcoma or congenital hemangiopericytoma, but the vast majority of cases are associated with KHE or TA, caused in at least large part by intra-tumoral platelet trapping. Untreated lesions do not regress. KHE is categorized as an "intermediate (locally aggressive)" soft tissue tumor by the WHO [48] due to rare reports of spread along (or perhaps multifocal involvement of) local lymphatic chains. True metastasis is unlikely, and no distant metastases have been reported.

Some KHE/TA are congenital, and most are reported in infants and young children under 5 years of age. Rarely, they arise in older children and adults. KMP is seen only in congenital/early infantile cases and not in all of those. Lesions vary from superficial locally infiltrative stains and plaques in the skin and subcutis to large masses in deep soft tissues. Typical locations include the extremities, the trunk, and the head and neck. They occasionally present as bulky body cavity or retroperitoneal masses and more rarely in the bone and spleen. On MRI they are usually diffusely enhancing, T2 hyperintense, with ill-defined margins that cross tissue planes.

Treatment options include a wide local excision, which is curative when feasible. Medical treatment is warranted for KMP, when the lesion is not resectable. Treatment of small lesions without KMP is controversial. No single medical treatment regimen has yielded consistent results. Vincristine is now the preferred treatment of choice. Interferon-alpha-2a and interferon-alpha-2b carry the risk of permanent spastic paraplegia. Corticosteroid monotherapy is not effective.

Histology

The typical histological features of KHE and TA overlap and often coexist in the same lesion, with those of TA commonly seen in superficial (cutaneous) aspects of a large mass in which classic features of KHE are seen more deeply. Classic KHE are infiltrative, ill-defined lesions with frequently coalescing nodules of spindled endothelial fascicles, which admix with nodular epithelioid nests and areas of more typical capillary formation (Fig. 1.16a). Lesional endothelial cells show

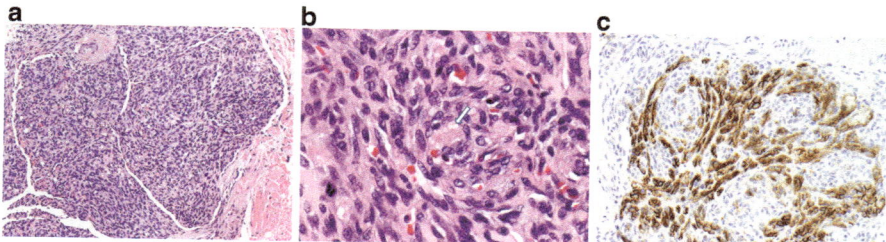

Fig. 1.16 Kaposiform hemangioendothelioma (KHE). (**a**) Infiltrative coalescing nodules of spindled endothelial cell fascicles admixed with epithelioid nests. (**b**) The spindle cells curve around pericyte-rich nests often containing a central platelet-rich microthrombus (*arrow*). (**c**) The spindled endothelial cells are strongly positive for podoplanin (shown) as well as CD34, CD31, LYVE-1, and PROX1

infrequent mitoses and are moderately plump, with eosinophilic to clear cytoplasm and bland nuclei. The component spindled cells form elongated slit-like lumina containing erythrocytes and curve around epithelioid nests rich in pericytes surrounding entrapped platelet-rich microthrombi (Fig. 1.16b). Hemosiderin deposition, red cell extravasation and fragmentation, and hyaline globules may be prominent. Dilated crescentic lymphatic vessels surround and intermingle with nodules, most prominently at margins of the lesion. Residual KHE lesions after successful medical treatment appear as dormant, often sclerotic, versions of the original disease process.

TA, as originally described in the dermatology literature, are composed of discrete lobules of capillaries that are scattered within the dermis and subcutis in a "cannonball" pattern. The intervening dermal stroma and subcutis are often fibrotic, but may be normal. The "cannonball" appearance is imparted by tightly condensed tumoral capillaries, often bulging into peripheral crescenting thin-walled vessels. Capillary pinpoint lumina may contain platelet microthrombi. Endothelial cells may be focally spindled, but less prominently than in KHE, lacking sweeping spindled cell fascicles and epithelioid nodules.

By immunohistochemical studies, spindled cells in KHE are positive for CD31 and CD34, variably weakly positive for vWF, and strongly positive for the lymphothelial markers podoplanin (D2-40), LYVE-1, and PROX1 (Fig. 1.16c) and negative for GLUT-1. Endothelial cells of TA may focally be positive for podoplanin, LYVE-1, and PROX1, but less extensively than lesional cells of KHE; they, too, are negative for GLUT-1 and other distinctive markers of IH. Platelet-rich microthrombi can be highlighted by immunostains for CD61 or CD31.

Pathogenesis

The significant degree of histological overlap between TA and KHE and the association of these two entities with KMP suggest that TA is a milder, more superficial form of KHE [59–64]. At a minimum, these lie at ends of a disease spectrum. The selective thrombocytopenia that characterizes KMP can be attributed at least in part to platelet trapping within KHE/TA vascular beds. Strong endothelial expression of lymphatic-associated antigens (Prox-1 and LYVE-1) and the blood vascular marker CD34 displayed by KHE supports the concept that these tumors, like Kaposi's sarcoma and a subset of angiosarcomas, have at least a partial lymphatic endothelial phenotype. This abnormal, mixed lymphatic–blood vascular phenotype may explain the propensity for platelet trapping [65]. Platelet transfusions, although sometimes clinically necessary, have in some cases paradoxically worsened KMP, suggesting that platelet activation within the tumor may amplify its growth by stimulating vascular proliferation [59], presumably by release of platelet-associated angiogenic agonists. A self-sustaining cycle of platelet trapping and tumor growth thus hypothetically may underlie the development of these lesions and KMP. Human herpes virus 8 sequences, characteristically present in Kaposi's sarcoma, have not been identified in KHE or TA; neither has been linked to HIV infection [62].

Multifocal Lymphangioendotheliomatosis with Thrombocytopenia (MLT)

Clinical Features

MLT is a relatively newly described, clinically and histologically distinctive vascular anomaly complicated by chronic mild-to-profound fluctuating thrombocytopenia and clinically significant gastrointestinal (GI) bleeding and/or pulmonary hemorrhage, particularly in infancy [65]. This entity has alternatively been termed congenital cutaneovisceral angiomatosis with thrombocytopenia, or CCAT [66]. It is not associated with the more severe level of thrombocytopenia seen in congenital KHE/TA. It occurs sporadically, with no clear racial or sexual predilection, as multiple congenital vascular lesions, with appearance of new lesions, slow progression of individual lesion, and no evidence of regression. Lesions are widely distributed in the skin, often with hundreds of lesions at birth, and in the viscera (gastrointestinal system, lungs, liver, spleen, and kidney), and in some cases in the bone, synovium, or muscle [67]. Skin lesions are flat or indurated, red-brown to burgundy, plaques or papules, often with central pallor or scaling, measuring up to a few centimeters in diameter. Clinically significant GI bleeding is near universally present and may be life-threatening. Partial GI resection is often needed for effective hemostasis. Medical treatment options have been reported to be of possible value in some, but not all cases.

Histology

Microscopically, lesions are composed of delicate vessels that are scattered throughout the tissue and lined by a monolayer of slightly hobnailed endothelial cells. Focally, endothelial cells line complex papillary projections that appear to float in the luminal plane of section (Fig. 1.17). Mitotic figures are rare to absent, though Ki-67 expression is increased (approximately 15 % of cells). By immunohistochemical studies, lesional endothelial cells are strongly positive for CD31, CD34, and LYVE-1 with light-to-absent positivity for podoplanin (D2-40) and negative for GLUT-1.

Pathogenesis

The pathogenesis of MLT is unknown, and it can be debated whether it represents a multifocal tumor or a multifocal vascular malformation. Its abnormal endothelial phenotype, with co-expression of lymphatic and blood vascular markers, suggests possible linkage to the associated selective thrombocytopenia, in analogy to the association between KHE/TA and KMP, but this remains purely speculative. Intuitively, it appears consistent with a multifocal vascular malformation syndrome. It is listed in the current ISSVA classification as a "provisionally unclassified vascular anomaly" [2]. It is currently not included in the WHO classifications.

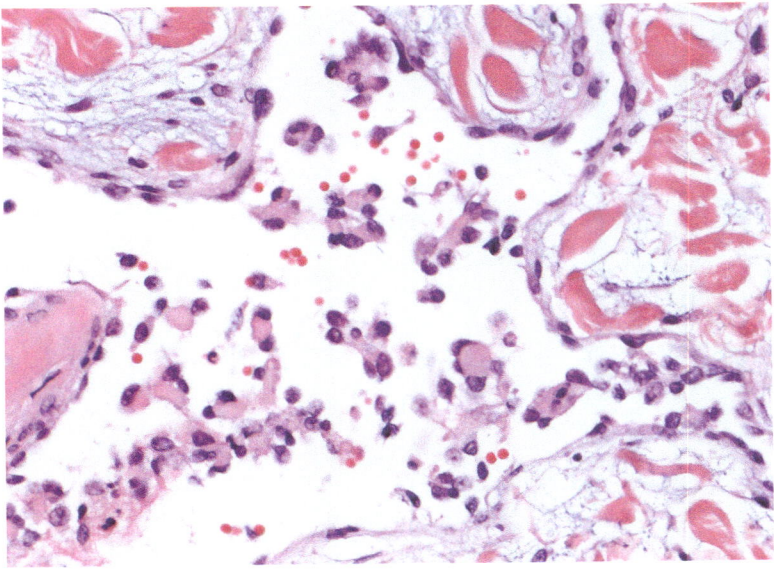

Fig. 1.17 Multifocal lymphangioendotheliomatosis with thrombocytopenia (MLT)

Intermediate (Rarely Metastasizing) Vascular Tumors

Papillary Intralymphatic Angioendothelioma (PILA)

Clinical Features

Often called *Dabska tumors*, these are rare subcutaneous and/or dermal lesions of highly distinctive histology and lymphatic differentiation [68, 69]. Many synonyms in addition to Dabska tumor have been applied to these tumors, including Dabska-type hobnail hemangioendothelioma [70] and malignant endovascular papillary angioendothelioma (by Dabska in 1969). Compilations of reported cases have shown no clear sex predilection, with approximately 75 % occurring in infants and children and the remainder in adults. Many reported cases have been congenital. These lesions are currently classified by the WHO as an intermediate (rarely metastasizing) vascular tumor [48] and are included in the 2014 ISSVA classification [2] as a locally aggressive or borderline tumor. Conservative excision with close follow-up is generally recommended; recurrences are common.

Histology

PILA is characterized by dermal/subcutaneous intercommunicating thin-walled vessels, lined by hobnail endothelial cells forming characteristic intraluminal papillary projections that focally show rosetting or matchstick-like patterns (Fig. 1.18),

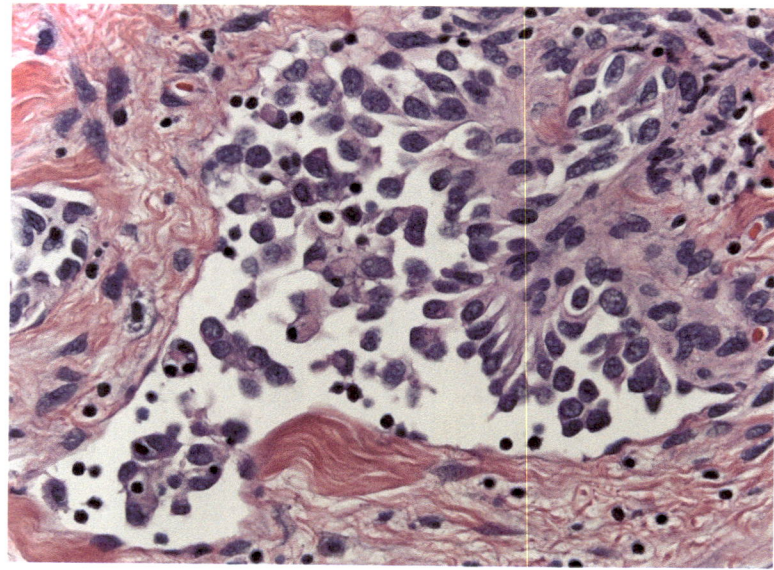

Fig. 1.18 Papillary intralymphatic angioendothelioma (PILA)

with immunoreactivity for lymphatic endothelial markers. Papillary projections display hyaline stromal cores and focally pericytes; lymphocytes typically cluster along the endothelial lining and infiltrate into the stroma.

Pathogenesis

Discussed with that of retiform hemangioendothelioma below.

Retiform Hemangioendothelioma

Clinical Features

Retiform hemangioendothelioma (RHE) is a rare neoplasm usually seen in young adults and sometimes children, in equal sex distribution, with very low potential for spread to local soft tissue or regional lymph nodes. It presents as a single nodule or multinodular plaque or exophytic tumor on the trunk or extremities, especially the distal lower extremities. Growth is slow, and there have been no tumor-related deaths. Optimal therapy is a wide excision with histologically clear margins. Otherwise, local recurrence is common.

Histology

Microscopic examination of RHE reveals diffuse infiltration of the dermis and/or subcutis by a poorly circumscribed, arborizing network of elongated thin-walled vessels forming a pattern reminiscent of normal rete testis and lined by hobnail-like endothelial cells that express CD34 as well as CD31. Mitotic figures are rare, and solid foci of spindle cells expressing endothelial markers are often present [71]. Dense lymphocytic infiltrates may be present, but the cavernous, lymphatic-like vessels and prominent intravascular proliferations of PILA (Dabska tumor) are lacking. Cytologic atypia is minimal, in contrast with well-differentiated angiosarcoma, which is the clinically most important differential for this entity and may have focal retiform architecture. Reports of expression of lymphatic endothelial markers such as podoplanin and Prox-1 in RE have been discordant [72]. A recent study demonstrated convincingly that RE endothelial cells usually do not express lymphatic markers such as podoplanin (D2-40) and VEGFR3 [73].

Pathogenesis

RHE is classified by the WHO as a vascular tumor of intermediate (rarely metastasizing) type [48] and by ISSVA as a locally aggressive or borderline vascular tumor [2]. When originally described by Calonje et al. [74] in 1994, it was interpreted as a low-grade angiosarcoma. Similarities in histology and clinical behavior to PILA (Dabska tumor), a tumor of well-documented lymphatic differentiation mainly affecting children led to a proposal that these two entities are biologically related and should be jointly described by the term *hobnail hemangioendothelioma*, with designation of *Dabska type* and *retiform type* [75], not to be confused with hobnail hemangioma (targetoid lymphatic malformation) discussed previously. However, the mounting evidence that RE endothelial cells, unlike those of PILA, usually do not express lymphatic markers has weakened this logic. There are no known genetic determinates; HHV-8 sequences were detected in one apparently immunocompetent patient's tumor [76].

Composite Hemangioendothelioma

Clinical Features

The term *composite hemangioendothelioma* (CHE) is used to describe rare vascular tumors classified by the WHO as of intermediate malignancy (rarely metastasizing) category [48] that are composed of varying mixtures of benign, low-grade malignant, and fully malignant vascular components. They usually arise in young adults, but one congenital case has been reported [77]. Most are in the skin and subcutis, often on the hands or feet, with variable, often nodular appearance [72]. The clinical course is protracted, and surgical excision is the usual treatment.

Recurrence is common, and sometimes multifocal, near the excision site [78, 79]. Three cases of metastasis have been reported, all of these to regional lymph nodes, with additional spread to adjacent skin in one case [78–80].

Histology

Tumors are composed of a complex mosaic of different patterns of benign and malignant vascular proliferation in variable proportions, most often including spindle cell hemangioma, retiform hemangioendothelioma, and epithelioid hemangioendothelioma [72]. Other reported components include PILA-like, kaposiform, and angiosarcoma-like patterns [78, 79, 81]. Borders are ill-defined, with lesional vessels infiltrating skin and subcutis.

Pathogenesis

Causality is unknown. This is an exceedingly rare entity with fewer than 30 cases reported. In these rare patients, lesions have occurred in association with chronic lymphedema (4 patients), "lymphangioma circumscriptum," arteriovenous malformation, and Maffucci syndrome (1 patient) [79, 81, 82]. One of the lymphedema-associated cases was radiation induced and included angiosarcoma-like foci, resembling a Stewart–Treves syndrome-like phenomenon [81]. Unlike Stewart–Treves syndrome, this case had an extremely protracted course in which the relatively indolent composite tumor arose 23 years post-radiation in the setting of long-term lymphedema and then progressed, as is typical of CHE, but not frank angiosarcoma, over several years before excision. The authors hypothesized that lymphedema and radiation might each have played a role in tumor development [81]. Importantly, recurrence and/or metastasis of CHE in reported cases appears unrelated to the presence or absence of angiosarcoma-like foci [81]. The compendium of evidence indicates that, biologically, CHE is not just a "low-grade" conventional angiosarcoma [81].

Malignant Vascular Tumors

Epithelioid Hemangioendothelioma

Clinical Features

Traditionally, the term *hemangioendothelioma* has denoted a vascular tumor of intermediate malignant potential; this has been the historical designation of *epithelioid hemangioendothelioma* (EHE), a relatively indolent tumor originally described by Weiss and Enzinger in 1982 that causes death in less than 50 % of patients with metastases. Approximately 30 % develop metastases in the regional nodes, lung, liver, or bone. EHE has more metastatic potential than other lesions classified as *hemangioendothelioma*, and the WHO and ISSVA have recently reclassified this entity as a malignant, rather than intermediate or borderline, vascular tumor. That classification is shared only with angiosarcoma [2, 48], although EHE is clearly characterized by better prognosis than classic angiosarcoma. EH typically occurs in adults, but in a younger age distribution than angiosarcoma. It is exceedingly rare in preadolescent children. Unlike angiosarcoma, women appear to be affected slightly more commonly than men. Mainline therapy is surgical excision with histologically clear margins without adjuvant chemotherapy or radiotherapy. Regional lymph nodes should be evaluated since they are a common metastatic site.

EHEs arise in the soft tissue, bone, skin, and various viscera, most typically presenting as a solitary, slightly painful, soft tissue mass, often on the extremities. Approximately 50 % of cases present multifocally [83]. Skin involvement is often associated with an underlying soft tissue or bone tumor, but entirely cutaneous examples occur. Multinodular cutaneous examples are reported and prompt consideration of possible metastasis from a visceral primary tumor [84]. Many are closely associated with or arise from a vessel, usually a vein. Occlusion of that vessel may be symptomatic, causing edema or thrombophlebitis. One study of 30 cases suggests that dermal tumors, most of these occurring on the extremities, may have a better prognosis than more deeply seated lesions [85].

Histology

EHE show an infiltrative growth pattern of epithelioid tumor cells with abundant pale eosinophilic cytoplasm forming poorly canalized nests and cords within a distinctive myxohyaline stroma. Cutaneous examples are generally well circumscribed and nodular and may be covered by hyperplastic epidermis [73]. An important clue to their endothelial origin is the presence of small intracytoplasmic vacuoles containing red blood cells (Fig. 1.19). Nuclei are usually vesicular with little or no atypia and contain small, inconspicuous nucleoli. In some cases, nuclear pleomorphism and mitotic figures are present. Mitotic rate is only weakly correlated with clinical outcome [83]. Inflammation is sparse, unlike epithelioid hemangioma (angiolymphoid hyperplasia with eosinophilia). The differential diagnosis includes epithelioid sarcoma, metastatic signet-ring adenocarcinoma, melanoma, and epithelioid angiosarcoma. An essential criterion is demonstration of endothelial differentiation with appropriate markers such as CD31 (most sensitive) and CD34. EHE also may be at least focally positive for podoplanin, Lyve-1, and Prox-1, suggesting lymphatic or mixed lymphatic–blood vascular differentiation [86, 87]. Ultrastructural studies show the EHE cells differ from normal endothelial cells in that they contain abundant cytoplasmic intermediate filaments [88]. These filaments can cause immunopositivity for cytokeratins and/or SMA, causing misdiagnosis [83, 89]. Histological differentiation of EHE from epithelioid angiosarcomas also may be problematic and relies upon recognition of the typical architectural pattern of EHE throughout the lesion, without the very atypical cells of epithelioid angiosarcoma that frequently demonstrate abnormal mitotic figures, apoptosis, and zonal necrosis.

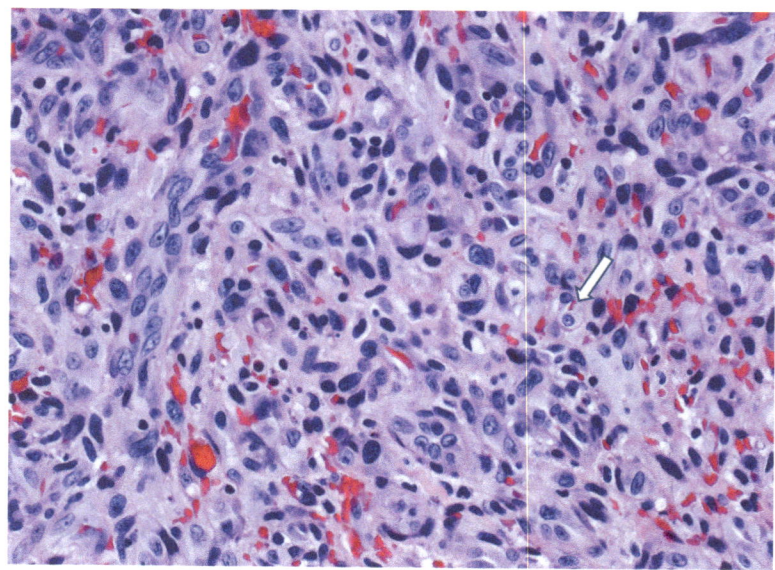

Fig. 1.19 Epithelioid hemangioendothelioma, characteristic intracytoplasmic vacuoles containing erythrocytes (*arrow*)

Pathogenesis

Most classical cases of EHE contain a t(1;3) (p36.3;q25) translocation that generates a *WWTR1-CAMTA1* fusion product that seems to be an early causative event in EHE oncogenesis [90–92]. *WWTR1* on 3q25 is involved in 14-3-3 transcriptional factor activation and signaling in the Hippo pathway that is highly expressed in normal endothelial cells [93]. *CAMTA1*, on 1p36, is one of a family of calmodulin-binding transcription factors normally found only in the brain. *CAMTA1* is likely a tumor suppressor gene since 1p36 is frequently lost in gliomas and neuroblastoma [94, 95].

Antonescu et al. recently reported a *WWTR1-CAMTA1* fusion-negative subset of EHE arising mainly in young adults that is morphologically distinguished from classical EHE by the presence of more well-developed vasoformative features and voluminous eosinophilic cytoplasm [96]. They subsequently identified an alternative gene fusion, *YAP1-TFE3* in this subset of EHE that is not found in classical *WWTR1-CAMTA1* fusion-positive EHE [96]. The transcriptional co-activator YAP1 shares sequence homology with WWTR1 and is a major downstream effector of the Hippo pathway [97]; TFE3 belongs to the MiT family of transcription factors; various TFE3 fusion partners associated with other tumor types, such as the *ASPL-TFE3* fusion in alveolar soft part sarcoma [98], are consistently expressed at a high level in the given tumor type, suggesting that TFE3 misexpression promotes tumorigenesis, likely by altering target gene expression [96]. Antonescu reported TFE3 protein expression, detected by immunohistochemistry, in all *WWTR1-CAMTA1* fusion-positive EHE cases examined, suggesting that this may be a useful screening method for detection of TFE3 rearrangements, especially when combined with CD31, Fli1, or ERG staining to help exclude other non-endothelial TFE3-positive neoplasms such as alveolar soft part sarcoma, PEComa, and Xp11-translocation positive renal cell carcinomas [96].

The *WWTR1-CAMTA1* and *YAP1-TFE3* fusions have not yet been detected in other neoplasms, in particular the morphologic mimics of EHE such as epithelioid angiosarcoma, epithelioid sarcoma-like HE, and epithelioid hemangioma, but it is not yet certain that they are unique to EHE [90, 91]. Both the *WWTR1-CAMTA1* and *YAP1-TFE3* fusion genes are reliably detected by fluorescence in situ hybridization and/or RT-PCR and thus have potentially important clinical diagnostic value [99]. Flucke et al. present data suggesting that TFE3 immunohistochemistry is of questionable reliability [99].

Angiosarcoma

Clinical Features

Angiosarcomas are rare neoplasms that usually occur in middle-age or older adults, more commonly in males, with highest incidence in those over 70 years of age. Clinical course is aggressive, with high mortality. It does occur exceedingly rarely in children and adolescents, accounting for approximately 0.3 % of pediatric sarcomas [100]. Rare examples that occur in childhood or adolescence are more likely to arise in or around viscera or in association with disease states such as chronic or congenital lymphedema and immunosuppression. In the pediatric age group, angiosarcomas are more likely to arise in or around viscera, with the heart and mediastinum the most common sites [101]. Among adults, the most common presentation is sun-exposed skin of the head and neck in an elderly patient, with strong predilection for Caucasians compared to individuals of African or Asian descent, and approximately a 2:1 predilection for males [102]. Prognosis is poor with a less than 15 % survival over a 5-year period [102]. Cutaneous angiosarcomas are also well described in the setting of chronic edema of any cause (Stewart–Treves syndrome) and sites of previous radiation therapy [103]. Cutaneous lesions in adults typically present as a bruise-like patch on the central face, forehead, or scalp which expands centrifugally, becomes violaceous, and develops elevated nodes that bleed. In contrast, pediatric cutaneous angiosarcomas are more common in females and on the lower extremity – they also tend to be small and unifocal [104].

Histology

Angiosarcomas are typically multinodular hemorrhagic masses. Necrosis and cystic degeneration are common. Those involving the skin do not vary in histology as a class between those of the "usual type" and those associated with chronic lymphedema or with chronic radiodermatitis. Variation in endothelial differentiation within

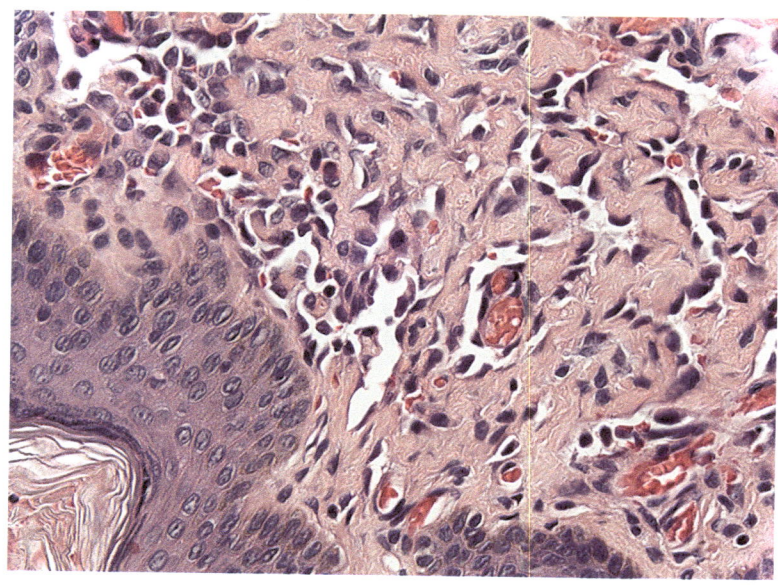

Fig. 1.20 Angiosarcoma, infiltrative pattern with moderate nuclear atypia

individual lesions is high. Well-differentiated areas display an anastomosing net-work of well-formed sinusoidal vessels, often bloodless, lined by a single layer of endothelial cells of slight to moderate nuclear atypia. These infiltrate between col-lagen bundles and groups of adipose cells (Fig. 1.20). In less well-differentiated vasoformative areas, pleomorphic endothelial cells with high mitotic rate pile up and form papillary projections. Poorly differentiated areas show solid areas without apparent lumen formation composed of high-grade spindled and epithelioid cells with abundant eosinophilic-to-amphophilic cytoplasm and large vesicular nuclei with prominent nucleoli, mimicking other high-grade sarcomas, carcinoma, or mela-noma. Tumors enriched in epithelioid cells are often called "epithelioid angiosarco-mas." Purely epithelioid cutaneous angiosarcomas are reported to be disproportionately high among pediatric cases (90 %) compared to adult ones (30 %) [105].

Most angiosarcomas immunoreact positively for typical endothelial markers such as CD31, CD34, and Fli1 [106–108], with CD31 generally considered most useful. A panel of antibodies is wise in light of differing sensitivities and specificity. Some examples show positivity for the lymphatic endothelial marker podoplanin [109, 110]. Immunohistochemical detection of factor VIII-related antigen (von Willebrand factor), although highly specific for endothelial cells, lacks sensitivity for vascular neoplasms and is negative or very weak even in well-differentiated angiosarcomas. Some angiosarcomas co-express endothelial markers and epithelial antigens such as EMA and AE1/3. This can lead to confusion with carcinoma, espe-cially in angiosarcomas with predominantly epithelioid cytology if not carefully considered [50]. Demonstration of coexistent CD31 expression is key.

Pathogenesis

Angiosarcomas are clonal proliferations of malignantly transformed cells expressing endothelial differentiation. Distinct upregulation of various vascular-specific receptor tyrosine kinase genes, including TIE1, KDR, TEK, and FLT1, has been observed in angiosarcomas compared with other sarcomas [111]. Furthermore, high-level MYC amplification on 8q24 is consistently seen in radiation-induced and lymphedema-associated angiosarcomas [112, 113]. MYC amplification has also been observed in a subset (breast and bone) of primary angiosarcomas [114]. MYC amplification is presumed to have a crucial role in angiosarcoma through upregulation of the miR-17-92 cluster, which downregulates thrombospondin-1, a potent inhibitor of angiogenesis [114]. It is potentially and diagnostically useful as well as mechanistically interesting that the WWTR1-CAMTA1 fusion typically seen in epithelioid hemangioendothelioma has not been detected in angiosarcoma, including epithelioid angiosarcoma [50].

Although sun-exposed skin of the head and neck is the most common site of adult angiosarcoma, cumulative sun exposure has not been shown definitively to be a predisposing factor. Human herpesvirus 8, strongly linked to Kaposi's sarcoma, also appears not to be associated with angiosarcoma. Environmental carcinogens linked to development of hepatic angiosarcoma include vinyl chloride, thorium dioxide (Thorotrast), and arsenic [115]. Angiosarcomas have been reported rarely in association with long-term exposure to various foreign materials [116], defunctionalized arteriovenous shunts in renal transplant patients [117], xeroderma pigmentosum [118], malignant germ cell tumors [119], neurofibromatosis, and Aicardi syndrome [120]. Radiation therapy-induced angiosarcomas without compounding lymphedema have also been well documented [121].

Convincing reported associations of angiosarcoma with benign vascular anomalies other than congenital lymphedema are vanishingly rare but include superimposition upon mixed lymphatic–venous malformation in one patient with Aicardi syndrome [122] and a few previously irradiated benign vascular lesions [123, 124] including one in a patient with Klippel–Trenaunay syndrome [125]. Historical reports of angiosarcoma arising in a port-wine stain are poorly documented; two examples (from 1990), and none since, are fairly convincing. Rossi and Fletcher found upon literature review in 2002 only 5 bona fide examples of spontaneous or radiation-induced angiosarcoma arising in benign vascular lesions and added 4 spontaneously arising cases (3 from AVMs and 1 from an intramuscular lesion) [126]. Hepatic angiosarcoma unresponsive to steroids or vincristine occurring coincidently with multiple cutaneous infantile hemangiomas has also been reported [127].

Mechanisms linking chronic lymphedema to development of angiosarcoma remain uncertain, although theories abound. Induction of neoplastic change by unknown carcinogens in accumulated lymphatic fluid has been suggested [128], as has the possibility that areas with chronic lymphedema are "immunologically privileged sites" due to loss of afferent lymphatic connections, allowing tumor cells to grow unchecked. It is often assumed that chronic lymphedema-associated angiosarcomas originate from lymphatics, explaining lymphatic-like histological features in some of these tumors, as well as a variable degree of reported expression of lymphatic markers. Growing data casts doubt on this assumption. Expression of the lymphatic endothelium-associated antigen VEGFR-3 was observed in 8 of 16 angiosarcomas in one series in which cases associated with lymphedema and prior irradiation were excluded [129]. Further, in another study, most angiosarcomas were found to co-express podoplanin and endothelial markers more typical of blood vessels, such as CD34 [109], suggesting that many angiosarcomas, independent of chronic edema setting, are of mixed lineage. Until this issue is further clarified, the use of the more generic term *angiosarcoma*, rather than *lymphangiosarcoma* or *hemangiosarcoma*, seems prudent.

Vascular Malformations

As congenital abnormalities in embryonic vascular morphogenesis, vascular malformations have limited postnatal endothelial mitotic activity. They are by definition present at birth (though may be hidden) and grow slowly and, in general, proportionately, as the child ages. They persist throughout life in continued relative mitotic quiescence. Like vascular tumors, the malformations are a heterogeneous group of clinicopathologically distinct entities of diverse, often still obscure etiology.

Histopathological distinction of vascular malformations from vascular tumors can at times be difficult, not only due to lack of clinical history, but also because the gross and microscopic appearances of vascular malformations tend to evolve postnatally and may include areas of vascular proliferation. Factors causing this evolution include progressive or intermittent vascular ectasia, recruitment of collateral vessels, organizing thrombosis, hormonal modulation, infection, scarring, and reactive neovascularization in response to abnormal intralesional hemodynamics or tissue ischemia. Despite these challenges, vascular malformations can usually be recognized as such. Correlation with clinical and radiological information is often helpful, if not essential.

Recent advances in our understanding of underlying pathogenetic mechanisms of several categories of familial and sporadic vascular malformations support increasingly precise classification and therefore more specifically targeted therapies. Vascular malformations may contain venous, capillary, lymphatic, or arterial components in any combination. Some forms are highly distinctive and easily recognized. Others are more diagnostically problematic. Accurate histopathological diagnosis is often required to guide effective therapy and meaningful research, complementing clinical and radiological evaluation. The pathologist's task is not only to subclassify these lesions per constituent vessel types and the presence or absence of increased endothelial mitotic activity, but to confirm or dispute the clinical and radiological impression; recognize patterns indicative or suggestive of specific subtypes that may have known genetic associations or predictable clinical behaviors; assess (for blood vascular malformations) histological evidence for stasis, high flow, or arteriovenous shunting; and advice the clinician regarding any indicated additional clinical laboratory and/or genetic testing. At a minimum, it can be very helpful to indicate what the lesion is not and what remains in the histological differential.

The current ISSVA-sanctioned classification of vascular anomalies, which can be downloaded at www.issva.org, stratifies vascular malformations first as "simple" or "combined" [2]. The "simple" malformations include (1) capillary malformations (CM), (2) lymphatic malformations (LM), (3) venous malformations (VM), and (4) arteriovenous malformations (AVM) and congenital arteriovenous fistulas (AVF). Subgroups have been added to each of the above groups, typically as genetic variants associated with specific types of lesions within each broader category have been recognized. The "combined" malformations, not surprisingly, are comprised of various clinically relevant mixtures of two or more "simple" malformations, specifically of CM, LM, VM, or AVM. Availability of the ISSVA classification is important to the field – firstly, because it was formulated and approved by a large multidisciplinary group of specialists in vascular anomalies and, secondly, because the current WHO classifications and current pathology textbooks do not yet adequately or accurately reflect the current state of knowledge and nosology in this field, certainly not for the malformations.

Summarized below are the key clinical features and current histopathological diagnostic criteria for each of the major categories of vascular malformations (CM, VM, AVM, and LM). Histological features of syndromic mixed VM-LM malformations and a short list of rare distinctive malformations with very recently recognized genetic determinants are also described. Omitted from discussion are malformations of the heart and major "named" conducting vessels, as well as the telangiectasias.

Capillary/Venulocapillary Malformations

The term *capillary malformation* (CM) encompasses a number of distinct clinico-pathological entities and yet still in this era of heightened nosologic awareness is used alone rather freely by pathologists and clinicians alike, often creating considerable confusion reflective of our still limited understanding. Care must be taken to provide, whenever possible, appropriate modifications of this term in order to clearly convey which type of "capillary malformation" is intended. Clinicians often use the term to refer to any clinically evident cutaneous vascular discoloration or "stain," a nonspecific phenomenon which can be associated with telangiectasias and arteriovenous, venous, and lymphatic malformations, with or without a true capillary malformative component. *Capillary malformations* (or often more properly *venulocapillary malformations*) do, as histologically well-characterized components, also occur as part of a number of complex syndromes, many of which causative gene defects have recently been identified.

The most common and well characterized of the capillary/venulocapillary malformations is the clinically and histologically distinctive cutaneous and sometimes deeper venulocapillary malformation known as facial "port-wine stain," caused by GNAQ somatic mutation [130]. This specific cutaneous vascular malformation, when combined with ipsilateral leptomeningeal and/or choroidal involvement, comprises *Sturge–Weber syndrome* [131]. Less common syndromes with still poorly described or understood capillary/venulocapillary components but known genetic associations include *CM-AVM* and *Parkes–Weber syndrome* (germline RASA1 mutations) [132], *Cowden's and Bannayan–Riley–Ruvalcaba syndromes* (germline PTEN mutations) [133], and *Klippel–Trenaunay syndrome* (somatic PIK3CA mutations) [134]. Lee et al. have recently proposed another entity to encompass cases of symmetrical tissue overgrowth with a vascular anomaly: *diffuse capillary malformation with overgrowth* [135], not yet histologically characterized. This proposed entity clinically falls outside of disorders with classical asymmetric overgrowth such as Klippel–Trenaunay syndrome. Also rising into the spotlight here is a rare, but long-recognized entity previously termed "verrucous hemangioma," which we designate *verrucous venulocapillary malformation*.

Cutaneous Capillary/Venulocapillary Malformations Caused by GNAQ Mutation (Port-Wine Stains)

This section focuses upon a sporadic, clinically distinctive, and well-recognized type of cutaneous venulocapillary malformation traditionally referred to by clinicians as *port-wine stain* (PWS). PWSs affecting the ophthalmic branch of the trigeminal nerve are often associated with venulocapillary abnormalities of the ipsilateral leptomeninges and eye, producing the neurocutaneous disorder known as *Sturge–Weber syndrome* (SWS). The strongly segmental pattern of PWS and Sturge–Weber syndrome has long suggested the probability of mosaicism due to somatic mutation of otherwise lethal genes. Very recently, the causative somatic mutation of the vast majority of cases of Sturge–Weber syndrome and nonsyndromic PWSs of the head and neck region was discovered – an activating nonsynonymous single nucleotide variant (c.548G → A, p.Arg183Gln) in the GNAQ gene [130]. Follow-up studies have confirmed this causative association and have also revealed rare linkage to somatic mutations at other nucleotides within the GNAQ gene sequence [136]. Pulsed-dye laser therapy lightens the stain.

Clinical Features

Port-wine stains are congenital, non-proliferative, non-involuting lesions but often become thickened and nodular over many years, secondary to progressive vascular ectasia, which begins superficially and extend to deeper vessels over time. They occur with equal sex predilection, in 0.3 % of all newborns, and usually affect the head and neck region [137–139]. Most are unilateral and segmental, but may be bilateral and/or multisegmental. Children born with a facial PWS have an approximately 6 % chance of having Sturge–Weber syndrome [138] with risk increased to 26 % when the PWS is located in the ophthalmic branch of the trigeminal nerve [139]. With Sturge–Weber syndrome, seizures and ocular complications (glaucoma) may arise. PWSs are cutaneous lesions, though some extend into the subcutis. Generalized soft tissue and/or bone hypertrophy is not uncommon in affected areas and may be extreme. Pyogenic granulomas may arise within PWS.

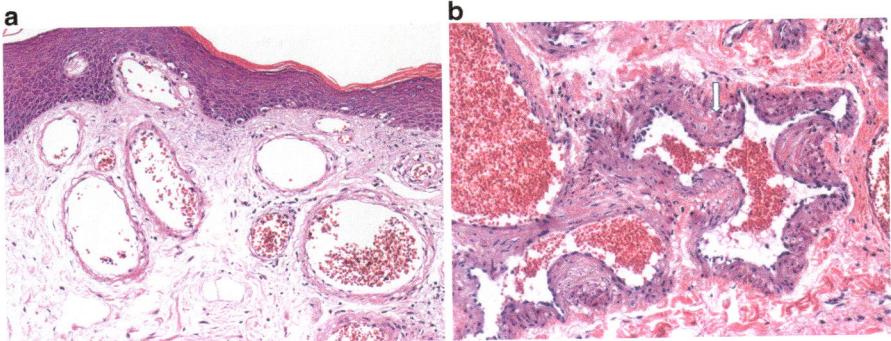

Fig. 1.21 Cutaneous port-wine stain (PWS), caused by somatic GNAQ mutation. (**a**) Dermal vessels of venulocapillary size progressively dilate without evidence of increased mitotic activity and little, if any, well-differentiated mural smooth muscle. (**b**) In cases complicated by soft tissue hypertrophy, vessels may develop thick coats of unusually plump smooth muscle (*arrow*)

Histology

PWSs are composed of dilated vessels of mature capillary or venular type. Vascular ectasia may not become prominent in histological sections until about 10 years of age, despite clinically evident red skin discoloration at birth. Dermal vessels of venulocapillary size progressively acquire a rounded dilated contour and are filled with blood, lined by thin endothelia associated with pericytes and occasionally a few well-differentiated smooth muscle cells, with no evidence of increased mitotic activity (Fig. 1.21a). The vascular wall becomes thickened and fibrotic over time. With generalized soft tissue hypertrophy, vessels may develop loosely organized thick coats of plump smooth muscle fibers (Fig. 1.21b) [140]. Gross nodule formation reflects focally exaggerated vascular ectasia and/or late development of complex epithelial, mesenchymal, and neural hamartomatous changes [141].

The vascular malformations affecting the brain of patients with Sturge–Weber syndrome are largely manifest in the leptomeninges ipsilateral to an associated cutaneous facial PWS and have been less rigorously studied than their cutaneous counterparts. As in the skin, the predominant vessels are dilated capillaries and venules (Fig. 1.22). Occasional dilated vessels may also be seen focally within the underlying cortex, typically accompanied by multiple foci of calcification and other reactive changes reflective of chronic seizure activity and altered blood flow.

Pathogenesis

Immunohistochemical evaluation of PWS for general endothelial and pericytic markers, basement membrane proteins, and fibronectin has not shown differences between normal skin and PWS [142]. Although it remains controversy as to whether dermal vessels are actually increased in number in PWS compared to normal skin [143, 144], there is no clear evidence that lesional vessel numbers change with time.

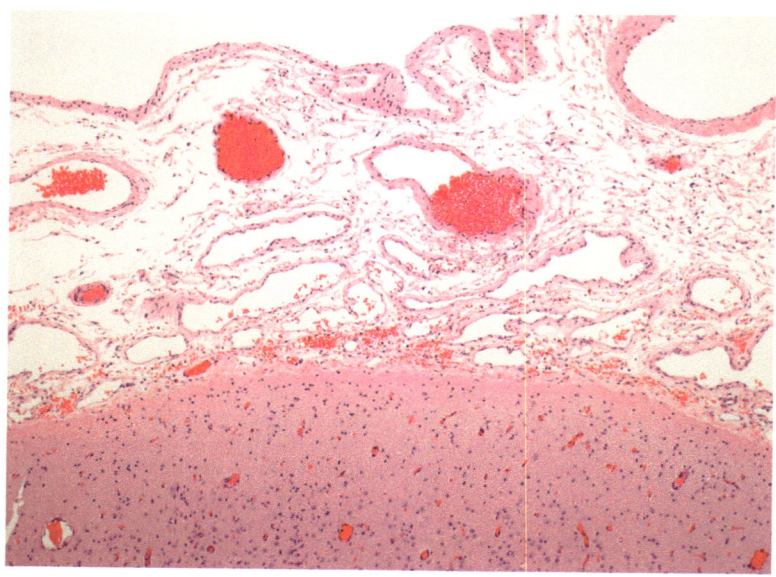

Fig. 1.22 Leptomeningeal venulocapillary malformation of Sturge–Weber syndrome (GNAQ mutation)

Studies employing S-100 immunostaining have reported a decrease in perivascular nerve density in PWS, suggesting that the progressive vascular dilatation character-istic of these lesions may be influenced by inadequate innervation [144, 145]. Observations of development of complex epithelial, mesenchymal, and neural hamartomatous changes in aged PWS have suggested genetically determined, mul-tilineage developmental field defect in the pathogenesis of this lesion [141].

The recent discovery by Shirley et al. [130] that a specific somatic mosaic activating mutation in GNAQ is associated with both the Sturge–Weber syndrome and non-syndromic port-wine stains is a game changer. GNAQ encodes Gαq, a member of the q class of G-protein alpha subunits that mediates signals between G-protein-coupled receptors and downstream effectors [130]. Shirley et al. have also shown that the somatic mosaic GNAQ encoding p.Arg183Gln amino acid substitutions in the skin and brain tissue from patients with the Sturge–Weber syndrome and in the skin tissue with nonsyndromic port-wine stains activates downstream MAPK signaling [130].

Activating mutations in genes encoding Gα subunits have previously been shown to be associated with a number of clinically important phenotypes, including the McCune–Albright syndrome [146], blue nevi and nevi of Ota [147], and uveal melanoma [147]. It is reasonable to conclude that the phenotypic effects of activating somatic GNAQ mutations would be determined by the specific cell lineages harboring or indirectly affected by the mutation as well as by the timing of the mutation during development and the degree of activation.

Venous Malformations

Clinical Features

Venous malformations are typically solitary lesions, localized or segmental, superficial or deep. Most are sporadic. Some present in association with complex syndromes and some are familial and multiple. Combination with lymphatic malformations is relatively common. By MRI, VMs are slow flow lesions, with low vascular resistance and bright hypersignal on T2-weighted spin echo. Superficial lesions enlarge over time due to increased venous pressure (increased by dependency or exertion). Common complications include chronic low-grade consumptive coagulopathy in large/extensive lesions and phleboliths and pain of unclear origin.

Histology

Endothelia of venous malformations are flattened and mitotically inactive. The vessel walls have no elastic interna and contain a variable amount of well-differentiated smooth muscle (usually scant relative to luminal diameter) (Fig. 1.23a). Vessels of capillary or venular proportions may also be present within the lesion. Disorganization of smooth muscle fibers may be seen. Dilated lumina are filled with red blood cells; luminal thrombi in various stages of organization, including calcified phleboliths, are often present, reflective of stasis (Fig. 1.23b). Organizing thrombi help distinguish these low-flow lesions from high-flow arteriovenous malformations. Recanalizing thrombi may show intravascular papillary endothelial hyperplasia (Masson's lesions, Masson's vegetant intravascular hemangioendothelioma). In early lesions, endothelial sprouts are seen to grow into fibrinous thrombus material, developing papillary fronds lined by a single layer of plump endothelial cells with no significant cytologic atypia. In later states, fibrin cores become collagenized and hyalinized, and endothelia attenuate. Lesional papillae fuse, resulting

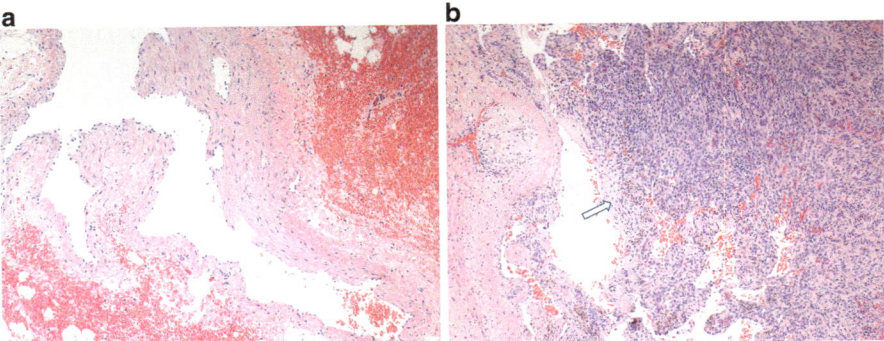

Fig. 1.23 Venous malformation (VM). (**a**) Lesional veins typically have relatively scant mural smooth muscle and are widely dilated or collapsed. (**b**) Due to stasis, organizing luminal thrombi are frequently present (*arrow*)

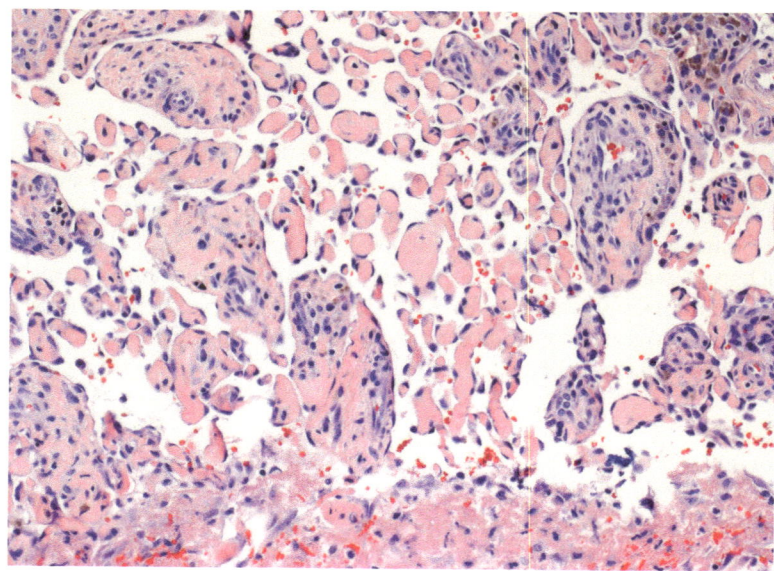

Fig. 1.24 Venous malformation, intravascular papillary endothelial hyperplasia (Masson's lesion). Organizing, recanalizing thrombus material may form complex papillary structures lined by endothelial cells, mimicking angiosarcoma

in an anastomosing meshwork of vessels, mimicking angiosarcoma, with without pleomorphism, necrosis or high mitotic activity (Fig. 1.24).

Pathogenesis

Multiple *mucocutaneous venous malformations* (VMCMs) (OMIM #600195) inherited as an autosomal dominant trait have been linked to a locus (*VMCM1*) on chromosome 9p21 and are caused by activating missense mutations in the TEK gene that encodes for endothelial cell-specific tyrosine kinase receptor TIE2, which binds angiopoietins [148, 149]. Formation of a VMCM lesion is thought to require loss at the second allele by somatic mutation, and an example of one such "second hit" has been identified [150]. This need for a second hit could explain why many inherited VMCM lesions appear in adolescence rather than at birth.

In more than half of inherited VMs, the detected TIE2 mutation is an Arg849 to tryptophan (R849W) substitution [149, 151]. More recent studies have also identified somatic TIE2 mutations in 85 % of sporadic VMs, although in these cases the mutation (L914F) leads to substitution of a leucine to a phenylalanine, producing a stronger TIE1-hyperphosphorylation effect than the inherited R849W mutation of VMCM [150, 152]. The L914F mutation of TIE2 in sporadic VM has not been identified in inherited cases and is likely lethal in germline. Sporadic VMs are present at birth and are typically solitary – new lesions do not appear over time. The mutated TIE2 receptors of inherited and sporadic VMs aberrantly activate AKT in a ligand-independent manner, causing decreased platelet-derived growth factor-B (PDGFB) production and secretion [153]. Since PDGFB is an important recruiter of mural cells, this may explain in part why the smooth muscle coats of VMs are irregular and attenuated [153].

Multiple venous malformations also occur in the poorly understood dysmorphic syndrome known as *blue rubber bleb nevus syndrome* (BRBNS), first described in 1958 by Bean [154]. Blue rubber bleb nevus syndrome comprises an association between multiple venous malformations of the skin and the gastrointestinal tract, complicated by gastrointestinal bleeding and anemia. Some cases of BRBNS are sporadic, and others autosomal dominant. Somatic *TIE2* mutations have also been identified in the majority of BRBNS patients but differ from the causative mutations of VMCM and common sporadic VM in that they occur as double cis-mutations on the same TIE2/TEK allele [155].

Verrucous Venulocapillary Malformation (Verrucous "Hemangioma")

This is a rare, but increasingly well-recognized, vascular anomaly that is a new addition to the rightful list of vascular malformations. Increasing well-recognized clinically and histologically, it is off the radar screen of the WHO and even in the last ISSVA classification is listed as a "provisionally unclassified vascular anomaly" [2]. Clinically and histologically it clearly best meets the criteria of a vascular malformation, rather than an intrinsically proliferative vascular tumor, despite having been labeled as a verrucous "hemangioma" in 1967 when it was originally described as such by Imperial and Helwig of the Armed Forces Institute of Pathology [156]. Even in that original paper, it was stated that "It is considered a vascular malformation, eg, a true structural variant of capillary hemangioma that secondarily develops reactive epidermal acanthosis, hyperkeratosis, and parakeratosis" – the use of the term "hemangioma" was merely a testament to generic use of that term for benign vascular lesions at that time. Mankani and Dufresne suggested in 2000 that the name be changed to verrucous [vascular] malformation [157], but that opinion has been resisted until very recently due to lingering uncertainty regarding the pathogenesis of these lesions and concerns that they might show evidence of cellular proliferation during their evolution [158]. Mulliken and Greene and colleagues have recently recommended the use of the term *verrucous venous malformation* [159]. We prefer designation as *verrucous venulocapillary malformation* congruent with the predominant nature of the component vessels.

Clinical Features

Verrucous venulocapillary malformations are striking congenital vascular anomalies that occur equally in males and females, presenting at birth as clinically distinctive, slightly raised singular, grouped, or confluent red-to-purple cutaneous lesions

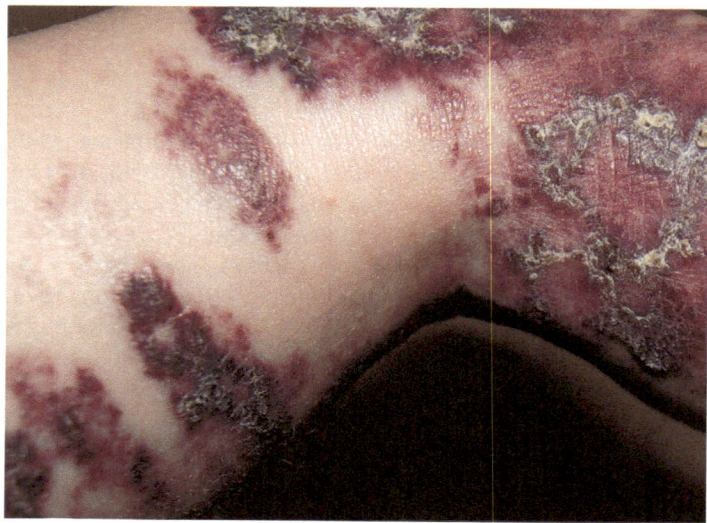

Fig. 1.25 Verrucous venulocapillary malformation, clinical. Singular, grouped, or confluent red-to-purple congenital lesions on the distal extremities that darken and become hyperkeratotic over time are typical. Photo courtesy of Beth Drolet

that upon microscopic examination have subcutaneous as well as superficial dermal components. The vast majority occur on the distal extremities, particularly the lower (Fig. 1.25). Rare examples have been reported on the trunk [160]. They progressively darken and become hyperkeratotic during childhood, often increasingly complicated by ulceration, bleeding, and scarring. They do not regress and are not associated with local tissue hypertrophy or other developmental anomalies.

Histology

Histological appearance varies with age and progressive secondary changes of epidermal orthotic hyperkeratosis and verrucous hyperplasia, but the persistent background lesion is one of dilated blood vessels, capillary or venular in type without coats of smooth muscle, populating the papillary dermis and occasionally the investing dermis around skin appendages. These spare the reticular dermis and appear again in the subcutis, usually smaller in caliber and often grouped, not infrequently showing intraluminal thrombi (Fig. 1.26a). The superficial dermal vessels are usually the most impressively dilated and focally raise the epidermis, expanding vascular papillae (Fig. 1.26b). Within the subcutis, dilated capillaries may cluster around nerve bundles. Lesional vessels consistently express endothelial markers of blood vascular differentiation, including CD31 and CD34. Focal positivity for lymphatic endothelial markers such as Prox-1 and podoplanin (D240) has been reported in some studies [161], but not others [162]. Mitotic activity is very low. Many verrucous venulocapillary malformations, as well as a few other

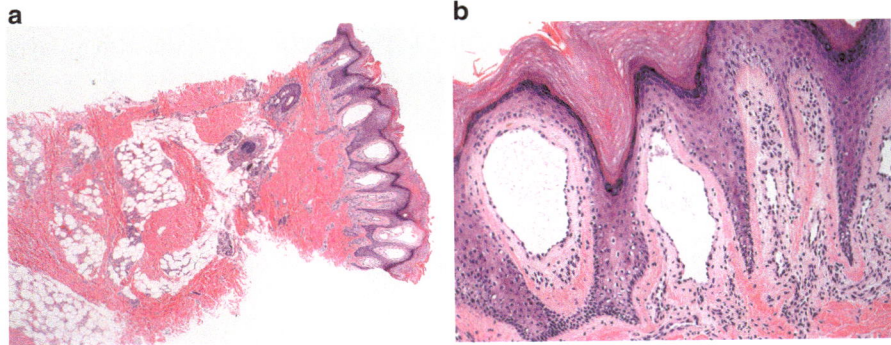

Fig. 1.26 Verrucous venulocapillary malformation, histology. (**a**) Low-power views show dilated capillaries and venules in the papillary dermis, sparing the reticular dermis, and appearing again in the subcutis. (**b**) The superficial vessels are dilated and expand dermal papillae; the epidermis becomes hyperkeratotic and verrucous, often ulcerating

capillary malformations, show light, focal immunoreactivity for GLUT1, paled by the intense endothelial GLUT1 positivity displayed by capillaries of the placenta and infantile hemangioma as part of a distinctive phenotype not seen in other vascular anomalies [17, 18]. Other markers of infantile hemangioma/placental capillaries, such as CD15 and indoleamine 2,3-dioxygenase, are not seen in verrucous malformations (P North, personal communication).

Pathogenesis

Verrucous venulocapillary malformations are vascular malformations, not tumors. Couto et al very recently reported the presence of a missense somatic mutation in mitogen-activated protein kinase kinase kinase 3 (MAP3K3) in 6 of 10 of these lesions at mutant allele frequencies ranging from 6 % to 19 % in affected tissue and did not find this mutant allele in unaffected tissue or in affected tissue from other types of vascular anomalies [159]. Since studies in MAP3k3 knockout mice have previously implicated MAP3K3 in vascular development, Map3K3 may cause verrucous venulocapillary (aka verrucous venous) malformations in humans [159].

Glomuvenous Malformations

Lesions characterized by the presence of benign glomus cells have been subclassified historically into categories such as diffuse type, solitary type, multiple type, solid type, adult type, and pediatric type. Current evidence supports division of these lesions into two major categories: (1) the glomus tumor proper, a cellular neoplasm that tends to be well circumscribed, solitary, and subungual, and (2) the so-called glomangioma, a frequently multifocal lesion, more properly termed *glomuvenous malformation*, that presents in infants or children and histologically resembles a venous malformation in which lesional vessels are surrounded by layers of glomus cells. The following discussion is restricted to this second category, which accounts for 10–20 % of all glomus cell lesions.

Clinical Features

Glomuvenous malformations (GVMs) are superficial lesions either present at birth or becoming evident in childhood or adolescence. They vary widely in phenotype from single punctate lesions to multiple, widely distributed to confluent, soft, red-to-blue nodules to large pink to deep blue plaques. Although clinically resembling venous malformations, GVMs tend to be bluer and more nodular or cobblestone-like in appearance, are less compressible, and do not swell with exercise or dependency [163]. There is no significant sex preponderance.

GVMs are less painful than the glomus tumor proper but may be tender to palpation, and attacks of pain may occur during menstruation and pregnancy. All reported cases have behaved in a benign fashion. Due to their more expansive, multifocal nature, GVMs are less amenable to surgery than common adult-type glomus tumors and may recur locally following subtotal resections and may progress locally [164]. Sclerotherapy is less effective for GVMs than for venous malformations [165].

Histology

GVMs consist of dilated, thin-walled veins in the dermis and subcutis, often distributed as separate nodules. They are histologically similar to those comprising venous malformations but are surrounded by one or more layers of cuboidal glomus cells (Fig. 1.27). The glomus cell component can be quite variable from region to region and vessel to vessel, making adequate sampling important. Like venous malformations without glomus cells, many GVMs contain organizing thrombi or phleboliths.

Pathogenesis

Some GVM are sporadic and in this case are always present at birth. At least 68 % of GVM, however, demonstrate an autosomal dominant pattern of inheritance [166, 167]. The inherited forms tend to be multiple and continue to appear later in life, sometimes in response to trauma [168]. Based on linkage disequilibrium studies of families with inherited GVM, a locus for GVM (termed GLMN) has been mapped to chromosome 1p21-p22 and encodes for a protein of still uncertain function termed glomulin [169–171]. The wide phenotypic variation in GVM, and variability of penetrance in affected families, has suggested possible important genotype–phenotype relationships. A recent study by Brouillard et al. of 162 families with GLMN mutation found 40 different mutations within the GLMN gene, the most frequent one present in

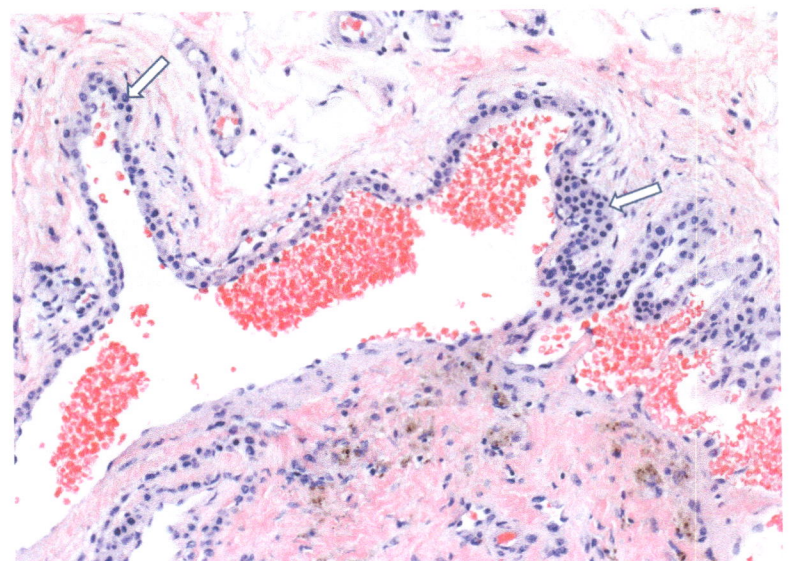

Fig. 1.27 Glomuvenous malformation. Component vessels are veins rimmed by one-to-several layers of bland, rounded glomus cells (*arrows*)

about 45 % of the families, without specific genotype–phenotype correlation and with a penetrance of 90 % [172]. Sporadic GVMs likely result from somatic mutations at this locus.

The high but incomplete penetrance, frequent multifocality, and delayed development of autosomal dominant inherited GVM have suggested the likelihood of second-hit somatic mutations in the pathogenesis of GVM. Amyere et al. investigated this possibility and found 16 somatic mutations, most of which were not intragenic, but rather were incidences of acquired uniparental isodisomy involving chromosome 1p13.1-1p12, a possible new fragile site [173]. Thus, as with inherited VMCM, familial GVM is inherited in a paradominant fashion, requiring a second-hit somatic mutation for lesion development.

The normal function of glomulin, also called FAP68, is still poorly understood. Pathways by which loss of glomulin/FAP68 function might affect GVM development are myriad and have been recently reviewed [155]. These possibilities include suggested glomulin interactions with hepatocyte growth factor and TGFβ signaling pathways [174, 175] and established binding of glomulin to the Rbx1 RING domain, leading to inhibition of the E3 ubiquitin ligase activity of the Cul1-RING1 ligase complex and thus affecting ubiquitination and degradation of various proteins such as cyclin E and c-Myc. Tron et al. recently demonstrated that glomulin deficiency is associated with increased levels of cyclin E and c-Myc [176]. In situ hybridization studies of mouse tissues demonstrate expression of glomulin in vascular smooth muscle cells during development [177].

Arteriovenous Malformations

Clinical Features

Most arteriovenous malformations (AVMs) occur sporadically as solitary lesions and may involve the skin and subcutis, soft tissue, bone, or viscera. Roughly half are obvious at birth, and most others become evident during early childhood as clinically significant arteriovenous shunting is recognized. Deep or intracranial lesions may not be apparent till later childhood or adulthood, particularly if shunting of low grade. AVM's progress over time, usually beginning in adolescence [178], as collateral arterial flow is recruited into the low-resistance vascular bed. On physical examination, those with superficial extension may raise the skin temperature and produce a palpable thrill or pulsation due to shunting. Common major complications include clinically significant, sometimes life-threatening, hemorrhage and local tissue ischemia due to arterial steal. AVMs often recur aggressively if incompletely excised or inadequately embolized.

Histology

Unlike AV fistulas, which are typically acquired lesions characterized by one or a few large AV shunts, sporadic AVMs are more complex developmental anomalies with a myriad, perhaps millions, of small abnormal AV connections that bypass a normally controlled, high-resistance vascular bed. Microscopic features vary widely from one area to another in the same lesion and between different lesions. Most histological sections show beds of arterioles, capillaries, and venules within a densely fibrous or fibromyxomatous background, intermixed with numerous larger-caliber arteries and thick-walled veins (Fig. 1.28a). In well-developed examples with high-grade shunting, the arteries are characteristically tortuous in contour and irregular in caliber, with thickened and fragmented elastic laminae. Component veins demonstrate changes reflective of elevated local venous pressure and turbulence, including irregular intimal and adventital fibrosis with irregularly thickened, focally fibrotic smooth muscle coats, often with intimal "bumpers" at points of venous tortuosity. Early AVM and those with lower-grade shunts will show more subtle findings. There is no evidence of thrombosis or intravascular papillary endothelial hyperplasia (which are typical of VM), consistent with the abnormally high venous flow and pressure of AVM. The actual AV shunts are difficult to impossible to find without extensive histological sectioning or special techniques.

Small vessel collections are a diagnostically important and variably prominent, sometimes dominant, component of AVM, varying widely in architecture between different lesions and within individual lesions. Many of these small vessel components are proliferatively active and enriched in plump capillaries that mimic, in some ways, a vascular tumor such as infantile hemangioma or "pyogenic granuloma." To be clear, these proliferations are negative for GLUT1 and in no way consistent with infantile hemangioma [15, 17]. Although often seen in deeply seated

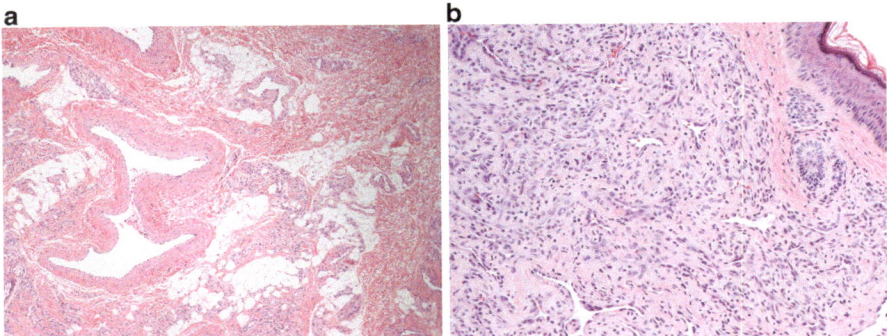

Fig. 1.28 Sporadic arteriovenous malformation (AVM), histology. (**a**) A complex combination of arterioles, capillaries, and venules is set within fibromyxoid stroma intermingled with larger-bore, often tortuous, arteries and thick-walled veins with reinforced mural structure in response to high flow. (**b**) Involved skin may show a ragged small vessel proliferation that lacks the delicate lobularity of IH

portions of AVM, particularly in skeletal muscle, scattered among larger-caliber arterial and venous components, these cellular small vessel proliferations are particularly prominent in ulcerated skin overlying and/or involved by AVM, producing a ragged "pseudokaposiform" proliferation of small vessels that lack the delicate lobularity of IH (Fig. 1.28b). This cutaneous phenomenon has traditionally been termed "Stewart–Bluefarb syndrome" [179] and is probably caused, at least in part, by tissue ischemia due to bypass of the normal capillary bed due to shunting.

AVMs and other high-flow vascular lesions associated with inherited syndromes and recently identified genetic defects overlap in histology with the much more common sporadic AVMs but display some distinctive features. These conditions include CM-AVM (capillary malformation–arteriovenous malformation) and Parkes–Weber syndrome [132], PTEN hamartoma tumor syndrome (PHTS) [133], and hereditary hemorrhagic telangiectasia (Rendu–Osler–Weber syndrome; HHT) [180, 181].

CM-AVM (OMIM #608354) is an inherited condition caused by RASA1 mutations and characterized by multiple small cutaneous vascular "stains" associated with AVMs/AVFs [132, 182]. The cutaneous stains of CM-AVM are small both histologically and clinically unlike other more common cutaneous capillary malformations. Grossly, they are often surrounded by a halo of pale skin, and they increase in number with age. Biopsies of these are so rare that few pathologists, even those specializing in vascular anomalies, have seen more than a handful. The histology has been described as minimally dilated capillaries in the dermis [183] and as subtle dilation of the superficial dermal microvasculature, with increase in small arteries and veins in the subcutis [184]. Given that these small cutaneous stains often demonstrate high flow upon Doppler examination, it has been suggested that these are a manifestation of an underlying AVM and not that of a capillary malformation [183]. The AVMs of CM-AVM are histologically similar to sporadic AVM (Fig. 1.29),

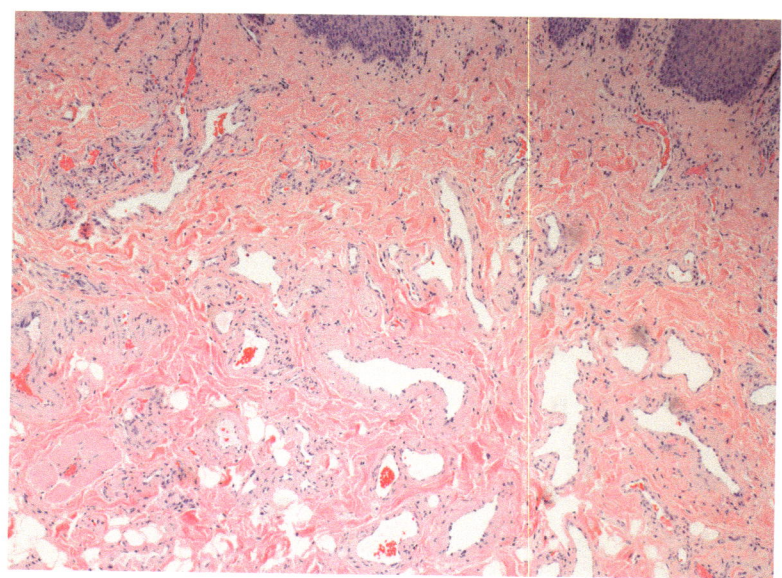

Fig. 1.29 AVM of CM-AVM, caused by RASA1 mutation

although less well documented. Reported examples have been located on the face or an extremity, intracranially, or intraspinally [182].

The vascular anomalies that arise as elements of PTEN hamartoma tumor syndromes are variable in histological content, but often contain a high-flow component with characteristic and visually peculiar features, including clusters of bizarre, thick-walled veins with concentrically fibrotic, muscular walls, honeycomb-like vascular complexes, tortuous small arteries, abundant fat and perivascular myxoid stroma, and hypertrophic nerves (Fig. 1.30).

The vascular lesions of HHT range from ectatic capillaries and venules in the skin and oral/nasal/gastrointestinal mucosa to prominent arteriovenous malformations and fistulas with dilated veins and arteries in the liver, lung, brain, and gastrointestinal tract [185].

Arterial embolization using polyvinyl alcohol or other foreign materials precedes most surgical resections of AVMs, in order to reduce intraoperative bleeding. This elicits a variable acute inflammatory response within the involved tissues. Tissue necrosis is a rare complication.

Pathogenesis

The vast majority of AVMs are sporadically occurring single lesions of unknown etiology. Approximately a third of CM-AVM patients with the cutaneous capillary malformations and pathognomonic heterozygous germline RASA1 mutations of

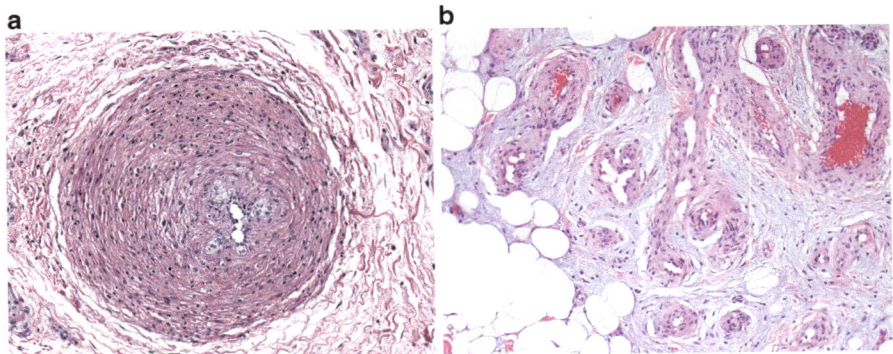

Fig. 1.30 PTEN-associated vascular hamartoma. Histology is highly variable, but characteristically includes peculiar thick-walled veins with concentrically fibrotic walls (**a**) and abundant perivascular myxoid stroma accompanying tortuous arteries (**b**). Other features include abundant fat, hypertrophic nerves, and honeycomb-like complexes of dilated thin-walled vessels (not shown)

this disorder also have fast-flow vascular lesions, either AVMs or arteriovenous fistulas (AVFs) [182]. These include approximately one-half of patients with Parkes–Weber syndrome, a condition that combines AVM, cutaneous CM, limb overgrowth, and sometimes LM [182]. Over 100 different RASA1 mutations have been identified in 132 CM-AVM families [132, 182, 186–188]. Most of these reported mutations result in premature stop codons, likely causing loss of function [132, 182]. In approximately one-third of patients with phenotypic findings equivalent to CM-AVM, RASA1 mutation has not been detected by applied methodologies, and about 25 % of cases are due to de novo RASA1 mutations [182].

Homozygous RASA1 knockout in mice is lethal at E9-9.5 due to severe vascular defects [189]. The multifocal nature and wide phenotypic variation of CM-AVM, with underlying germline RASA1 loss in one allele, could be explained by need for a second-hit somatic mutation to complete local loss of RASA1 function, precipitating development of a focal vascular lesion. Evidence to support that possibility has been reported for one patient [182]. The specific mechanism by which RASA1 loss causes CM-AVM lesions is unclear. RASA1 encodes for the small cytoplasmic molecule p120RasGAP, which negatively modulates the Ras signal transduction pathway by activating the Ras GTPase activity, thus helping convert Ras into its inactive ADP-bound form. Thus, loss of RASA1 function through mutation would be expected to result in Ras signaling overactivity in response to stimulation by growth factors/hormones/cytokines that act through the Ras signaling pathway. Since the vascular lesions of CM-AVM are focal and likely require a second-hit mutation to cause lesion development, the timing of that second hit during vascular development, and the specific cell types that harbor the second hit, would be expected to be important variables in resultant phenotypic expression. RASA1 mutations have also been implicated in basal cell carcinoma [190], and somatic mutations in RAS gene isoforms are frequent in cancer, but increased risk of malignancy in CM-AVM has not been observed [182].

Lymphatic abnormalities, in addition to CM-AVM, have been reported in human patients with germline RASA1 abnormalities and in RASA1 knockout/knockin mice [191, 192]. In mice, RASA1 maintains the lymphatic vasculature in a quiescent state [193]. Kawasaki et al. have presented evidence that RASA1 suppresses endothelial mTORC1 activity within the EPHB4 signaling pathway [194].

HHT, also known as Osler–Rendu–Weber syndrome, is an autosomal dominant disorder characterized by multisystemic angiodysplasia leading to frequent epitaxis, telangiectasias, GI bleeding, and arteriovenous shunts in the liver, brain, and lung. It has been linked to mutations in two genes and has therefore been designated HHT type 1 (HHT1; gene, *ENG*; chromosome 9q34.1) and HHT type 2 (HHT2; gene, *ACVRL1*, chromosome 12q11-q14) [195, 196]. HHT in association with juvenile polyposis has been linked to mutations in *SMAD4* [197]. ENG encodes for endoglin, a co-receptor of the TGFβ (beta) family, whereas *ACVRL1* encodes ALK1, a type 1 receptor of the TGFβ (beta) family; SMAD4 encodes a transcription factor critical for TGFβ (beta) signaling [198]. Recently, BMP9 loss of function mutations has been casually linked to a vascular-anomaly syndrome with phenotypic overlap with hereditary hemorrhagic telangiectasia [199]. BMP9 and BMP10 are bone morphogenetic proteins that are circulating growth factors of the TGFβ family that have been shown to bind directly with high affinity to ALK1 and endoglin; both are thought to help maintain endothelial cells in a quiescent state that is dependent on the level of ALK1/endoglin activation in endothelial cells [198]. Tillet and Bailly have hypothesized that a deficient BMP9/BMP10/ALK1/endoglin pathway may lead to reactivation of angiogenesis or a greater sensitivity to an angiogenic stimulus, resulting in endothelial hyperproliferation and hypermigration that could lead to vasodilatation and generation of an AVM [198].

The mechanisms by which germline PTEN mutations in PHTS produce vascular malformations are poorly understood. The tumor suppressor gene PTEN encodes for a dual-specificity phosphatase that antagonizes the phosphoinositol-3-kinase (PI3K)/Akt pathway, leading to G1 cell cycle arrest and/or apoptosis and also inhibits cell spreading via the focal adhesion kinase pathway [200].

Lymphatic and Mixed Lymphatic–Venous Malformations

Clinical Features

Lymphatic malformations (LMs) have traditionally been referred to as "lymphangiomas," despite general absence of significant endothelial mitotic activity. Just as blood vascular malformations are presumed to be developmental errors in morphogenesis of the blood vasculature, LMs are thought to be errors in morphogenesis of the lymphatic vascular system. Relatively superficial LMs are usually evident at birth or within in the first year or two of life. In addition to the more common presentations in the skin and subcutis, LM may also involve deeper soft tissues, bone, or viscera and may not become evident until older childhood or later. They can be localized or regional and may diffusely involve many tissue planes or organ systems.

In current practice it has been found to be useful to subclassify LM as either macrocystic, microcystic, or combined. Macrocystic LMs, defined arbitrarily by a cyst diameter of at least 0.5 cm, have traditionally been termed "cystic hydromas." Microcystic LMs are more common and may develop anywhere. Macrocystic LMs most commonly occur in the loose connective tissue of the neck, axilla, chest wall, or groin and often change in size due to progressive distention of the lymphatic spaces by lymph fluid. LMs often enlarge with systemic or local infection. Surgical excision of macrocystic LM has significant morbidity, and a mainstay of therapy has become sclerotherapy with irritants such as killed bacteria (OK-432) or doxycycline [201, 202]. Combined microcystic and macrocystic LMs are common. Treatment of microcystic and combined microcystic–macrocystic LM is problematic; sclerotherapy for these is generally ineffective.

LMs are often associated with significant soft tissue (particularly fat) and bony overgrowth. LMs involving the superficial skin or mucosae typically form fragile, clear surface vesicles that often ulcerate or bleed and become dark. Many dermal or mucosal lymphatic malformations are associated with more deeply seated lesions composed of larger vessels, explaining the frequent recurrence of resected dermal lesions. Upper airway obstruction is a significant risk in LM involving the tongue or oropharynx. Chylous ascites/intestinal lymphangiectasia or pleural or pericardial effusions may complicate abdominal and thoracic LM.

Generalized lymphatic anomaly (GLA), often called "lymphangiomatosis," is an extensive LM involving viscera and/or bone, often with coincident involvement of the skin or soft tissues. The spleen, liver, lung, and intestine are commonly involved viscera. Clinical morbidity is high due to the lung involvement, effusions, and bone erosion and fracture.

The close relationship between the lymphatic and venous systems during embryonic development may explain why some low-flow malformations include both lymphatic and venous and/or capillary components. Lesions from patients with Klippel–Trenaunay syndrome (KTS) and related disorders most consistently exemplify this phenomenon, but solitary mixed malformations of lymphatic, venous, and capillary vessels are also commonly observed in nonsyndromic patients. KTS envelops a spectrum of complex, segmental congenital disorders characterized by a variable combination of lymphatic and capillary–venous malformations associated with skeletal and adipose tissue overgrowth in the involved segment [6, 203].

Histology

Microcystic LMs are comprised by dilated small vessels with angular-to-rounded contours lined by a single layer of flattened-to-slightly hobnailed endothelial cells, rimmed by rare pericytes and little or no smooth muscle (Fig. 1.31a). These are filled with clear fluid and sometimes a few lymphocytes and/or macrophages. Traumatized lymphatic vessels may contain abundant erythrocytes. In microcystic LMs involving skin or mucosa, the dilated lymphatic vessels often protrude into superficial vascular papillae, causing bleb formation and epidermal/mucosal

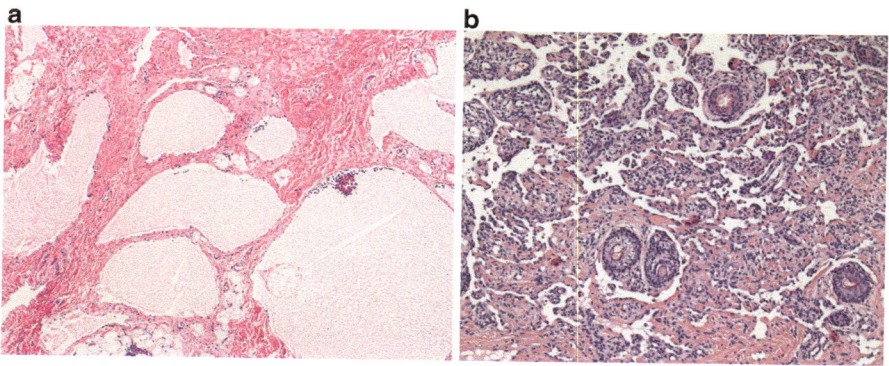

Fig. 1.31 Lymphatic malformations (LM), predominately microcystic. (**a**) Component vessels are dilated and rounded-to-angular in shape, filled with proteinaceous fluid and often a few lymphocytes and/or macrophages. Vessel walls are composed of flattened-to-slightly hobnailed endothelial cells associated with a few pericytes. (**b**) Some examples are more infiltrative, ramifying among and between tissue elements

hyperplasia. Overlying epidermis may appear hyperkeratotic and verrucous, and the surrounding stroma may be fibrotic and chronically inflamed. The vessels of diffusely infiltrative microcystic LMs often wrap extensively around tissue structures, producing the appearance of free-floating tissue elements and a complex anastomosing vasculature reminiscent of lymphangiosarcoma (Fig. 1.31b). Focal lymphoendothelial spindling and hyperplasia may be evident in some of the lesional vessels of these diffuse LMs. A low but appreciable level of proliferative activity indicated by cell cycle markers such as Ki-67 may be present.

Macrocystic LM vessels have thicker, irregular coats of smooth muscle and/or fibrous tissue and may have valves. Vessel lumina usually contain proteinaceous material and a few lymphocytes and/or macrophages. In many LMs, the enlarged lumina contain abundant blood or organizing myxoid thrombus material resulting from vessel wall injury or communication with the venous system. This makes it difficult to distinguish veins from lymphatics and may suggest a venous or mixed venous–lymphatic malformation. This distinction can usually be made by immunoreaction for antigens such as podoplanin (with the D2-40 antibody) or PROX1 that are expressed by lymphatic endothelial, but not blood vascular endothelial cells (Fig. 1.32). Care in interpretation must be taken, however, since the endothelial cells of larger lymphatic vessels may show spotty or even absent staining for lymphatic endothelial markers. The surrounding stroma often shows a lymphocytic infiltrate varying from a few scattered cells to striking, organoid aggregates containing lymphoid follicles.

Gorham–Stout disease, aka "disappearing bone disease," is a form of GLA characterized by prominent, typically multifocal intraosseous LM. The affected bones undergo cystic cortical osteolysis due to progressively dilated intraosseous lymphatic spaces, resulting in "disappearance" of bones in imaging studies, particularly plain film. Histologically, dilated, extremely thin-walled lymphatic vessels that may be extremely difficult to appreciate in routine sections expand the marrow

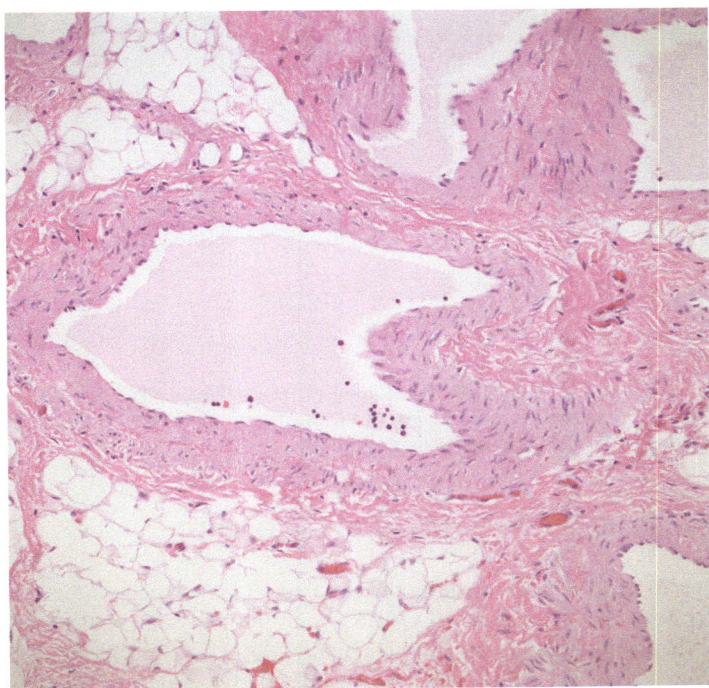

Fig. 1.32 Lymphatic malformation, mixed macrocystic and microcystic. The walls of larger lymphatic vessels may contain substantial smooth muscle

space, compressing and eventually thinning the cortical bone, sometimes to the point of pathological fracture. Immunohistochemistry for the pan-endothelial marker CD31 is useful to identify the endothelial lining of the cystically dilated spaces, and immunohistochemistry for podoplanin confirms lymphatic differentiation (Fig. 1.33). In many patients with multifocal bony involvement by LM, viscera (especially spleen) are also affected by LM. Periosseous extension into soft tissue is common. Rare cases of osteolysis with similar but localized clinical and radiological presentation may be associated with VM or AV fistula instead of LM.

Some spontaneously aborted fetuses with posterior cervical swellings traditionally referred to as "cystic hydroma" have been shown to have increased cutaneous lymphatics (e.g., trisomy 13 and 21), whereas those with monosomy X (Turner's syndrome) do not show increased or dilated lymphatics [204].

The histology of KTS is generally typical of VM and LM, with variably distributed components of each. Overlying areas of cutaneous involvement compounded by reaction to expansion of dermal papillae by ectatic capillaries or lymphatics create a PWS-like surface stain punctuated by angiokeratoma-like lesions. Eccrine glands are often notably enlarged and surrounded by myxoid stroma. Veins may demonstrate striking mural smooth muscle disarray. The malformations are largely cutaneous and subcutaneous but may also infiltrate deep skeletal muscle. Subcutaneous fat is increased.

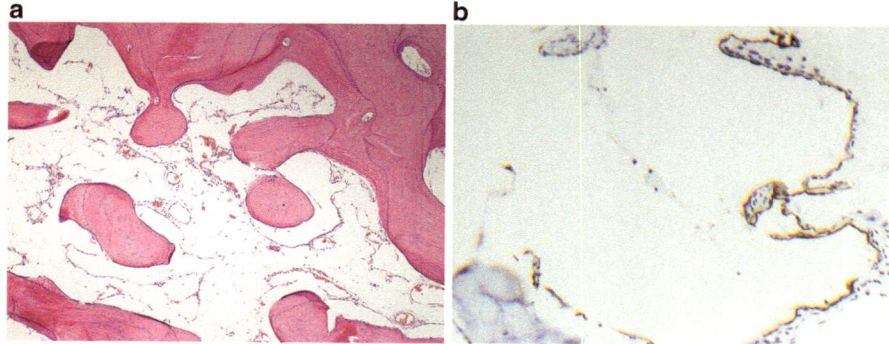

Fig. 1.33 Intraosseous LM (Gorham–Stout disease). The dilated, fragile lymphatic vessels are often difficult to see in routine H&E-stained histological sections and can be highlighted usefully with immunostains for CD31 (**a**) and podoplanin (**b**)

Pathogenesis

Several malformative/overgrowth syndromes that often include lymphatic malformations as a component, such as CLOVES syndrome and KTS, have recently been linked to activating mutations in phosphatidylinositol-4,5-bisphosphate 3-kinase, catalytic subunit alpha (*PIK3CA*), which encodes the catalytic subunit of the enzyme phosphatidylinositol 3-kinase (PI3K) [134, 205–207]. Importantly, somatic *PIK3CA* mutations were also found in 16/17 cases of isolated LM, occurring at low frequency (<10 %) in the affected tissue, determined by highly sensitive droplet digital PCR for 5 common *PIK3CA* mutations [134]. This latter study did not include matched normal tissues (e.g., blood) in the mutational analysis. Activating *PIK3CA* mutations also occur frequently in human cancer [208] where they enhance tumor growth in the setting of other oncogenic mutations [209]. It is not yet clear if *PIK3CA* mutation alone can produce LM or whether additional genetic or environmental influences are necessary. Specific *PIK3CA* mutations have not correlated with the specific phenotype of the various disorders characterized by *PIK3CA* mutations [134]. As with somatic mutations in other genes and other groups of disorders, influential factors intuitively would include developmental stage at the time of somatic mutation, cell type and location within the embryo of the originally mutated cell, and pluripotent or multipotent potential of the mutated cell population.

References

1. Mulliken JB, Glowacki J. Hemangiomas and vascular malformations in infants and children: a classification based on endothelial characteristics. Plast Reconstr Surg. 1982;69:412–22.
2. Wassef M, Blei F, Adams D, Alomari A, Baselga E, Berenstein A, Burrows P, Frieden IJ, Garzon MC, Lopez-Gutierrez J-C, Lord DJE, Mitchel S, Powell J, Prendiville J, Vikkula M. Vascular anomalies classification: recommendations from the international society for the study of vascular anomalies. Pediatrics, originally published online 8 June 2015; doi: 10.1542/peds.2014-3673

3. Bowers RE, Graham EA, Thominson KM. The natural history of the strawberry nevus. Arch Dermatol. 1960;82:667–70.
4. Powell TG, West CR, Pharoah PO, Cooke RW. Epidemiology of strawberry haemangioma in low birthweight infants. Brit J Dermatol. 1987;116:635–41.
5. Waner M, Suen JY. The natural history of hemangiomas. In: Waner M, Suen JY, editors. Hemangiomas and vascular malformations of the head and neck. New York: Wiley; 1999. p. 13–45.
6. Mulliken JB, Fishman SJ, Burrows PE. Vascular anomalies. Curr Probl Surg. 2000;37: 519–84.
7. Huang SA, Tu HM, Harney JW, Venihaki M, Butte AJ, Kozakewich HP, Fishman SJ, Larsen PR. Severe hypothyroidism caused by type 3 iodothyronine deiodinase in infantile hemangiomas. N Engl J Med. 2000;343(3):185–9.
8. Waner M, North PE, Scherer K, Frieden I, Mihm M. The non-random distribution of facial hemangiomas. Arch Dermatol. 2003;139:869–75.
9. Metry DW, Haggstrom AN, Drolet BA, et al. A prospective study of PHACE syndrome in infantile hemangiomas: demographic features, clinical findings, and complications. Am J Med Genet Part A. 2006;140A:975–86.
10. Drolet BA, Dohil M, Golomb MR, et al. Early stroke and cerebral vasculopathy in children with facial hemangiomas and PHACE association. Pediatrics. 2006;117(3):959–64.
11. Iacobas I, Burrows PE, Frieden IJ, Liang MG, Mulliken JB, Mancini AJ, Kramer D, Paller AS, Silverman R, Wagner AM, Metry DW. LUMBAR: association between cutaneous infantile hemangiomas of the lower body and regional congenital anomalies. J Pediatr. 2010;157(5):795–801.e1-7. doi:10.1016/j.jpeds.2010.05.027. Epub 2010 Jul 2.
12. Leaute-Babreze C, Dumas de la Roque E, Hubiche T, et al. Propranolol for severe hemangiomas of infancy. NEJM. 2008;358(24):2649–51.
13. Drolet BA, Frommelt PC, Chamlin SL, Haggstrom A, Bauman NM, Chiu YE, Chun RH, Garzon MC, Holland KE, Liberman L, MacLellan-Tobert S, Mancini AJ, Metry D, Puttgen KB, Seefeldt M, Sidbury R, Ward KM, Blei F, Baselga E, Cassidy L, Darrow DH, Joachim S, Kwon EK, Martin K, Perkins J, Siegel DH, Boucek RJ, Frieden IJ. Initiation and use of propranolol for infantile hemangioma: report of a consensus conference. Pediatrics. 2013;131(1):128–40. doi:10.1542/peds.2012-1691. Epub 2012 Dec 24.
14. Mawn LA. Infantile hemangioma: treatment with surgery or steroids. Am Orthopt J. 2013;63:6–13.
15. North PE, Waner M, Buckmiller L, James CA, Mihm MC. Vascular tumors of infancy and childhood: beyond capillary hemangioma. Cardiovasc Pathol. 2006;15:303–17.
16. North PE. Vascular tumors and malformations of infancy and childhood. Pathol Case Rev. 2008;13(6):213–35.
17. North PE, Waner M, Mizeracki A, et al. Jr. GLUT1: a newly discovered immunohistochemical marker for juvenile hemangiomas. Hum Pathol. 2000;31:11–22.
18. North PE, Waner M, Mizeracki A, et al. A unique microvascular phenotype shared by juvenile hemangiomas and human placenta. Arch Dermatol. 2001;137:559–70.
19. Ritter MR, Dorrell MI, Edmonds J, Friedlander SF, Friedlander M. Insulin-like growth factor 2 and potential regulators of hemangioma growth and involution identified by large-scale expression analysis. Proc Natl Acad Sci. 2002;99:7455–60.
20. Blei F, Walter J, Orlow SJ, et al. Familial segregation of hemangiomas and vascular malformations as an autosomal dominant trait. Arch Dermatol. 1998;134:718–22.
21. Walter JW, Blei F, Anderson JL, et al. Genetic mapping of a novel familial form of infantile hemangioma. Am J Med Genet. 1999;82:77–83.
22. Cheung DS, Warman ML, Mulliken JB. Hemangioma in twins. Ann Plast Surg. 1997;38: 269–74.
23. Barnes C, Huang S, Kaipainen A, et al. Evidence by molecular profiling for a placental origin of infantile hemangioma. PNAS. 2005;102:19097–102.
24. Ritter MR, Butschek RA, Friedlander M, et al. Pathogenesis of infantile hemangioma: new molecular and cellular insights. Exp Rev Mol Med. 2007;9:1–19.
25. North PE, Waner M, Brodsky MC. Are infantile hemangiomas of placental origin? Ophthalmology. 2002;109:633–4.

26. Kleinman ME, Tepper OM, Capla JM, et al. Increased circulating AC133+ CD34+ endothelial progenitor cells in children with hemangioma. Lymphat Res Biol. 2003;1(4):301–7.
27. Yu Y, Flint AF, Mulliken JB, Wu JK, Bischoff J. Endothelial progenitor cells in infantile hemangioma. Blood. 2004;103(4):1373–5.
28. Khan ZA, Boscolo E, Picard A, et al. Multipotential stem cells recapitulate human infantile hemangioma in immunodeficient mice. J Clin Invest. 2008;118(7):2592–9.
29. Dadras SS, North PE, Bertoncini J, Mihm MC, Detmar M. Infantile hemangiomas are arrested in an early developmental vascular differentiation state. Mod Pathol. 2004;17(9):1068–79.
30. Jinnin M, Medici D, Park L, Limaye N, et al. Suppressed NFAT-dependent VEGFR1 expression and constitutive VEGFR2 signaling in infantile hemangioma. Nat Med. 2008;14(11): 1236–46.
31. Munabi NC, Tan QK, Garzon MC, Behr GG, Shawber CJ, Wu JK. Growth hormone induces recurrence of infantile hemangiomas after apparent involution: evidence of growth hormone receptors in infantile hemangioma. Pediatr Dermatol. 2015;1–5.
32. North PE, Waner M, James CJ, et al. Congenital nonprogressive hemangioma: a distinct clinicopathological entity unlike infantile hemangioma. Arch Dermatol. 2001;137:1607–20.
33. Enjolras O, Mulliken JB, Boon LM, et al. Noninvoluting congenital hemangioma: a rare cutaneous vascular anomaly. Plast Reconstr Surg. 2001;107:1647–54.
34. Berenguer B, Mulliken JB, Enjolras O, et al. Rapidly involuting congenital hemangioma: clinical and histopathologic features. Pediatr Dev Pathol. 2003;6:495–510.
35. Nasseri E, Piram M, McCuaig CC, Kokta V, Dubois J, Powell J. Partially involuting congenital hemangiomas: a report of 8 cases and review of the literature. J Am Acad Dermatol. 2014;70(1):75–9.
36. Gorincour G, Kokta V, Rypens F, Garel L, Powell J, Dubois J. Imaging characteristics of two subtypes of congenital hemangiomas: rapidly involuting congenital hemangiomas and noninvoluting congenital hemangiomas. Pediatr Radiol. 2005;35(12):1178–85.
37. DeAos I, James CA, North PE. Hepatic "hemangioma": not a singular entity. Abstracts, 15th international congress on vascular anomalies, Wellington, NZ, 23 Feb 2004, p. 12.
38. Paltiel HJ, Burrows PE, Kozakewich HPW, et al. Solitary infantile hemangioma: a distinct clinicopathological entity. Abstracts, 15th international congress on vascular anomalies, Wellington, NZ, 23 Feb 2004, p. 12.
39. Christison-Lagay ER, Burrows PE, Alomari A, et al. Hepatic hemangiomas: subtype classification and development of a clinical practice algorithm and registry. J Pediatr Surg. 2007; 42:62.
40. Hsi Dickie B, Fishman SJ, Azizkhan RG. Hepatic vascular tumors. Semin Pediatr Surg. 2014;23(4):168–72.
41. Huang SA, Tu HM, Harney JW, Venihaki M, Butte AJ, Kozakewich HP, Fishman SJ, Larsen PR. Severe hypothyroidism caused by type 3 iodothyronine deiodinase in infantile hemangiomas. NEJM. 2000;343(3):185–9.
42. Al Dhaybi R, Lam C, Hatami A, Powell J, McCuaig C, Kokta V. Targetoid hemosiderotic hemangiomas (hobnail hemangiomas) are vascular lymphatic malformations: a study of 12 pediatric cases. J Am Acad Dermatol. 2012;66:116–20.
43. Mentzel T, Partanen TA, Kutzner H. Hobnail hemangioma ('targetoid hemosiderotic hemangioma'): clinicopathologic and immunohistochemical analysis of 62 cases. J Cutan Pathol. 1999;26:279–86.
44. Franke FE, Steger K, Marks A, Kutzner H, Mentzel TJ. Hobnail hemangiomas (targetoid hemosiderotic hemangiomas) are true lymphangiomas. J Cutan Pathol. 2004;31(5):362–7.
45. Olsen TG, Helwig EB. Angiolymphoid hyperplasia with eosinophilia. A clinicopathologic study of 116 patients. J Am Acad Dermatol. 1985;12:781–96.
46. Nielsen GP, Srivastava A, Kattapuram S, et al. Epithelioid hemangioma of bone revisited. A study of 50 cases. Am J Surg Pathol. 2009;33:270.
47. Fetsch JE, Weiss S. Observations concerning the pathogenesis of epithelioid hemangioma (angiolymphoid hyperplasia with eosinophilia). Mod Pathol. 1991;4:449.

48. Fletcher CDM, Bridge JA, Hogendoorn PCW, Mertens F. WHO classification of soft tissue tumours. In: WHO classification of tumours of soft tissue and bone, 4th edn. Lyon: IARC Press; 2013. p. 11.
49. Antonescu C. Malignant vascular tumors – an update. Mod Pathol. 2014;27:S30–8.
50. Weiss SW, Enzinger FM. Spindle cell hemangioendothelioma. A low-grade angiosarcoma resembling a cavernous hemangioma and Kaposi's sarcoma. Am J Surg Pathol. 1986;10: 521–30.
51. Perkins P, Weiss SW. Spindle cell hemangioendothelioma. An analysis of 78 cases with reassessment of its pathogenesis and biologic behavior. Am J Surg Pathol. 1996;20: 1196–204.
52. Fletcher CD. Vascular tumors: an update with emphasis on the diagnosis of angiosarcoma and borderline vascular neoplasms. Monogr Pathol. 1996;38(Chapter 6):181–206.
53. Fletcher CD, Beham A, Schmid C. Spindle cell haemangioendothelioma: a clinicopathological and immunohistochemical study indicative of a non-neoplastic lesion. Histopathology. 1991;18:291–301.
54. Imayama S, Murakamai Y, Hashimoto H, Hori Y. Spindle cell hemangioendothelioma exhibits the ultrastructural features of reactive vascular proliferation rather than of angiosarcoma. Am J Clin Pathol. 1992;97:279–87.
55. Fukunaga M, Ushigome S, Nikaido T, et al. Spindle cell hemangioendothelioma: an immunohistochemical and flow cytometric study of six cases. Pathol Int. 1995;45:589–95.
56. Amyere M, Dompmartin A, Wouters V, Enjolras O, Kaitila I, Docquier P-L, Godfraind C, Mulliken JB, Boon LM, Vikkula M. Common somatic alterations identified in Maffucci syndrome by molecular karyotyping. Mol Syndromol. 2014;5:259–67.
57. Pansuriya TC, van Eijk R, d'Adamo P, van Ruler MA, Kuijjer ML, Oosting J, Cleton-Jansen AM, van Oosterwijk JG, Verbeke SL, Meijer D, van Wezel T, Nord KH, Sangiorgi L, Toker B, Liegl-Atzwanger B, San-Julian M, Sciot R, Limaye N, Kindblom LG, Daugaard S, Godfraind C, Boon LM, Vikkula M, Kurek KC, Szuhai K, French PJ, Bovée JV. Somatic mosaic IDH1 and IDH2 mutations are associated with enchondroma and spindle cell hemangioma in Ollier disease and Maffucci syndrome. Nat Genet. 2011;43(12):1256–61.
58. Schaap FG, Frech PJ, Bovée JV. Mutations in the isocitrate dehydrogenase genes IDH1 and IDH2 in tumors. Adv Anat Pathol. 2013;20:32–8.
59. Enjolras O, Wassef M, Mazoyer E, Frieden IJ, Rieu PN, Drouet L, Taieb A, Stalder JF, Escande JP. Infants with Kasabach–Merritt syndrome do not have "true" hemangiomas. J Pediatr. 1997;130:631–40.
60. Zukerberg LR, Nickoloff BJ, Weiss SW. Kaposiform hemangioendothelioma of infancy and childhood. An aggressive neoplasm associated with Kasabach-Merritt syndrome and lymphangiomatosis. Am J Surg Pathol. 1993;17:321–8.
61. Niedt GW, Greco MA, Wieczorek R, et al. Hemangioma with Kaposi's sarcoma-like features: report of two cases. Pediatr Pathol. 1989;9:567–75.
62. Lyons LL, North PE, Mac-Moune Lai F, et al. Kaposiform hemangioendothelioma: a study of 33 cases emphasizing its pathologic, immunophenotypic, and biologic uniqueness from juvenile hemangioma. Am J Surg Pathol. 2004;28(5):559–68.
63. Enjolras O, Mulliken JB, Wassef M, et al. Residual lesions after Kasabach-Merritt phenomenon in 41 patients. J Am Acad Dermatol. 2000;42:225–35.
64. Le Huu AR, Jokinen CH, Ruben BP, Mihm M, Weiss SW, North PE, Dadras SS. Expression of Prox1, lymphatic endothelial nuclear transcription factor, in kaposiform hemangioendothelioma and tufted hemangioma. Am J Surg Pathol. 2010;34(11):1563–73.
65. North PE, Kahn T, Cordisco MR, et al. Multifocal lymphangioendotheliomatosis with thrombocytopenia: a newly recognized clinicopathological entity. Arch Dermatol. 2004;140:599–606.
66. Prasad V, Fishman SJ, Mulliken JB, et al. Cutaneovisceral angiomatosis with thrombocytopenia. Pediatr Dev Pathol. 2005;8:407–19.
67. Maronn M, Catrine K, North PE, et al. Expanding the phenotype of multifocal lymphangioendotheliomatosis with thrombocytopenia. Pediatr Blood Cancer. 2009;52(4):531–4.

68. Fanburg-Smith JC, Michal M, Partanen TA, et al. Papillary intralymphatic angioendothelioma (PILA): a report of twelve cases of a distinctive vascular tumor with phenotypic features of lymphatic vessels. Am J Surg Pathol. 1999;23:1004–10.
69. Fanburg-Smith JC. Papillary intralymphatic angioendothelioma. In: Fletcher CDM, Bridge JA, Hogendoorn PW, Mertens F, editors. WHO classification of tumors of soft tissue and bone. Lyon: IARC Press; 2013. Chap. 8, p. 148.
70. Goldblum JR, Folpe AL, Weiss SW. Hobnail (Dabska-retiform) hemangioendothelioma. In: Enzinger and Weiss's soft tissue tumors, 6th edn. Philadelphia: Elsevier Saunders; 2014. p. 693–8.
71. Sangüeza OP, Requena L. Malignant neoplasms. In: Pathology of vascular skin lesions. Totowa: Humana Press; 2003. Chap. 9, p. 217–74.
72. Requena L, Kutzner H. Hemangioendothelioma. Semin Diagn Pathol. 2013;30:29–44.
73. Parsons A, Sheehan DJ, Sangueza OP. Retiform hemangioendotheliomas usually do not express D2-40 and VEGFR-3. Am J Dermatopathol. 2008;30:31–3.
74. Calonje E, Fletcher CD, Wilson-Jones E, Rosai J. Retiform hemangioendothelioma. A distinctive form of low-grade angiosarcoma delineated in a series of 15 cases. Am J Surg Pathol. 1994;18:115–25.
75. Weiss SW, Goldblum JR. Enzinger and Weiss's soft tissue tumors, 4th edn. St. Louis: Mosby; 2001.
76. Schommer M, Herbst RA, Brodersen JP, et al. Retiform hemangioendothelioma: another tumor associated with human herpesvirus 8? J Am Acad Dermatol. 2000;42:290–2.
77. Reis-Filho JS, Paiva ME, Lopes JM. Congenital composite hemangioendothelioma: case report and reappraisal of the hemangioendothelioma spectrum. J Cutan Pathol. 2002;29(4):226–31.
78. Requena L, Luis Díaz J, Manzarbeitia F, Carrillo R, Fernández-Herrera J, Kutzner H. Cutaneous composite hemangioendothelioma with satellitosis and lymph node metastases. J Cutan Pathol. 2008;35(2):225–30.
79. Nayler SJ, Rubin BP, Calonje E, Chan JK, Fletcher CD. Composite hemangioendothelioma: a complex, low-grade vascular lesion mimicking angiosarcoma. Am J Surg Pathol. 2000; 24(3):352–61.
80. Aydingöz IE, Demirkesen C, Serdar ZA, Mansur AT, Yaşar S, Aslan C. Composite haemangioendothelioma with lymph-node metastasis: an unusual presentation at an uncommon site. Clin Exp Dermatol. 2009;34(8):e802–6.
81. McNab PM, Quigley BC, Glass LF, Jukic DM. Composite hemangioendothelioma and its classification as a low-grade malignancy. Am J Dermatopathol. 2013;35(4):517–22.
82. Fukunaga M, Suzuki K, Saegusa N, Folpe AL. Composite hemangioendothelioma: report of 5 cases including one with associated Maffucci syndrome. Am J Surg Pathol. 2007;31(10): 1567–72. PMID: 17895759.
83. Lau K, Massad M, Pollak C, Rubin C, Yeh J, Wang J, Edelman G, Yeh J, Prasad S, Weinberg G. Clinical patterns and outcome in epithelioid hemangioendothelioma with or without pulmonary involvement: insights from an internet registry in the study of a rare cancer. Chest. 2011;140(5):1312–8. PMID: 21546438.
84. Vignon-Pennamen MD, Varroud-Vial C, Janssen F, Degott C, Verola O, Cottenot F. Cutaneous metastases of hepatic epithelioid hemangioendothelioma. Ann Dermatol Venereol. 1989;116(11): 864–6. French. PMID: 2619191.
85. Mentzel T, Beham A, Calonje E, et al. Epithelioid hemangioendothelioma of skin and soft tissues: clinicopathologic and immunohistochemical study of 30 cases. Am J Surg Pathol. 1997;21:363–74.
86. Miettinen M, Wang ZF. Prox1 transcription factor as a marker for vascular tumors-evaluation of 314 vascular endothelial and 1086 nonvascular tumors. Am J Surg Pathol. 2012;36(3):351–9.
87. Naqvi J, Ordonez NG, Luna MA, Williams MD, Weber RS, El-Naggar AK. Epithelioid hemangioendothelioma of the head and neck: role of podoplanin in the differential diagnosis. Head Neck Pathol. 2008;2(1):25–30.
88. Vasquez M, Ordóñez NG, English GW, Mackay B. Epithelioid hemangioendothelioma of soft tissue: report of a case with ultrastructural observations. Ultrastruct Pathol. 1998;22(1): 73–8.

89. Quante M, Patel NK, Hill S, et al. Epithelioid hemangioendothelioma presenting in the skin: a clinicopathologic study of eight cases. Am J Dermatopathol. 1998;20:541–6.

90. Tanas MR, Sboner A, Oliveira AM, Erickson-Johnson MR, Hespelt J, Hanwright PJ, Flanagan J, Luo Y, Fenwick K, Natrajan R, Mitsopoulos C, Zvelebil M, Hoch BL, Weiss SW, Debiec-Rychter M, Sciot R, West RB, Lazar AJ, Ashworth A, Reis-Filho JS, Lord CJ, Gerstein MB, Rubin MA, Rubin BP. Identification of a disease-defining gene fusion in epithelioid hemangioendothelioma. Sci Transl Med. 2011;3(98):98.

91. Errani C, Zhang L, Sung YS, Hajdu M, Singer S, Maki RG, Healey JH, Antonescu CR. A novel WWTR1-CAMTA1 gene fusion is a consistent abnormality in epithelioid hemangioendothelioma of different anatomic sites. Genes Chromosomes Cancer. 2011;50(8):644–53. PMID: 21584898.

92. Mitelman F, Johansson B, Mertens F. The impact of translocations and gene fusions on cancer causation. Nat Rev Cancer. 2007;7(4):233–45. PMID: 17361217.

93. Chan SW, Lim CJ, Chen L, et al. The Hippo pathway in biological control and cancer development. J Cell Physiol. 2011;226:928–39.

94. Attiyeh EF, London WB, Mosse YP, et al. Chromosome 1p and 11q deletions and outcome in neuroblastoma. N Engl J Med. 2005;353:2243–53.

95. Barbashina V, Salazar P, Holland EC, et al. Allelic losses at 1p36 and 19q13 in gliomas: correlation with histologic classification, definition of a 150-kb minimal deleted region on 1p36, and evaluation of CAMTA1 as a candidate tumor suppressor gene. Clin Cancer Res. 2005;11:1119–28.

96. Antonescu CR, Le Loarer F, Mosquera JM, Sboner A, Zhang L, Chen CL, Chen HW, Pathan N, Krausz T, Dickson BC, Weinreb I, Rubin MA, Hameed M, Fletcher CD. Novel YAP1-TFE3 fusion defines a distinct subset of epithelioid hemangioendothelioma. Genes Chromosomes Cancer. 2013;52:775–84.

97. Dong J, Feldman G, Huang J, Wu S, Zhang N, Comerford SA, Gayyed MF, Anders RA, Maitra A, Pan D. Elucidation of a universal size-control mechanism in Drosophila and mammals. Cell. 2007;130(6):1120–33.

98. Ladanyi M, Lui MY, Antonescu CR, Krause-Boehm A, Meindl A, Argani P, Healey JH, Ueda T, Yoshikawa H, Meloni-Ehrig A, Sorensen PH, Mertens F, Mandahl N, van den Berghe H, Sciot R, Dal Cin P, Bridge J. The der(17)t(X;17)(p11;q25) of human alveolar soft part sarcoma fuses the TFE3 transcription factor gene to ASPL, a novel gene at 17q25. Oncogene. 2001;20:48–57.

99. Flucke U, Vogels RJ, de Saint Aubain Somerhausen N, Creytens DH, Riedl RG, van Gorp JM, Milne AN, Huysentruyt CJ, Verdijk MA, van Asseldonk MM, Suurmeijer AJ, Bras J, Palmedo G, Groenen PJ, Mentzel T. Epithelioid hemangioendothelioma: clinicopathologic, immunhistochemical, and molecular genetic analysis of 39 cases. Diagn Pathol. 2014;9:131. PMID: 24986479.

100. Ferrari A, Casanova M, Bisogno G, Cecchetto G, Meazza C, Gandola L, Garaventa A, Mattke A, Treuner J, Carli M. Malignant vascular tumors in children and adolescents: a report from the Italian and German Soft Tissue Sarcoma Cooperative Group. Med Pediatr Oncol. 2002;39:109–14. PMID: 12116058.

101. Deyrup AT, Miettinen M, North PE, Khoury JD, Tighiouart M, Spunt SL, Parham D, Weiss SW, Shehata BM. Angiosarcomas arising in the viscera and soft tissue of children and young adults: a clinicopathologic study of 15 cases. Am J Surg Pathol. 2009;33:264–9. PMID: 18987547.

102. Holden CA, Spittle MF, Jones EW. Angiosarcoma of the face and scalp, prognosis and treatment. Cancer. 1987;59:1046–57.

103. Brenn T, Fletcher CD. Radiation-associated cutaneous atypical vascular lesions and angiosarcoma: clinicopathologic analysis of 42 cases. Am J Surg Pathol. 2005;29:983–96.

104. Deyrup AT, Miettinen M, North PE, Khoury JD, Tighiouart M, Spunt SL, Parham DM, Shehata BM, Weiss SW. Pediatric cutaneous angiosarcomas: a clinicopathologic study of 10 cases. Am J Surg Pathol. 2011;35:70–5.

105. Deyrup AT, McKenney JK, Tighiouart M, Folpe AL, Weiss SW. Sporadic cutaneous angiosarcomas: a proposal for risk stratification based on 69 cases. Am J Surg Pathol. 2008;32:72–7.

106. Folpe AL, Chand EM, Goldblum JR, Weiss SW. Expression of Fli-1, a nuclear transcription factor, distinguishes vascular neoplasms from potential mimics. Am J Surg Pathol. 2001;25:1061–6. PMID: 11474291.
107. DeYoung BR, Swanson PE, Argenyi ZB, Ritter JH, Fitzgibbon JF, Stahl DJ, Hoover W, Wick MR. CD31 immunoreactivity in mesenchymal neoplasms of the skin and subcutis: report of 145 cases and review of putative immunohistologic markers of endothelial differentiation. J Cutan Pathol. 1995;22:215–22.
108. Miettinen M, Lindenmayer AE, Chaubal A. Endothelial cell markers CD31, CD34, and BNH9 antibody to H- and Y-antigens – evaluation of their specificity and sensitivity in the diagnosis of vascular tumors and comparison with von Willebrand factor. Mod Pathol. 1994;7(1):82–90. PMID: 7512718.
109. Breiteneder-Geleff S, Soleiman A, Kowalski H, Horvat R, Amann G, Kriehuber E, Diem K, Weninger W, Tschachler E, Alitalo K, Kerjaschki D. Angiosarcomas express mixed endothelial phenotypes of blood and lymphatic capillaries: podoplanin as a specific marker for lymphatic endothelium. Am J Pathol. 1999;154:385–94. PMID: 10027397.
110. Kahn HJ, Bailey D, Marks A. Monoclonal antibody D2-40, a new marker of lymphatic endothelium, reacts with Kaposi's sarcoma and a subset of angiosarcomas. Mod Pathol. 2002; 15:434–40.
111. Antonescu CR, Yoshida A, Guo T, Chang NE, Zhang L, Agaram NP, Qin LX, Brennan MF, Singer S, Maki RG. KDR activating mutations in human angiosarcomas are sensitive to specific kinase inhibitors. Cancer Res. 2009;69:7175–9. PMID: 19723655.
112. Manner J, Radlwimmer B, Hohenberger P, Mössinger K, Küffer S, Sauer C, Belharazem D, Zettl A, Coindre JM, Hallermann C, Hartmann JT, Katenkamp D, Katenkamp K, Schöffski P, Sciot R, Wozniak A, Lichter P, Marx A, Ströbel P. MYC high level gene amplification is a distinctive feature of angiosarcomas after irradiation or chronic lymphedema. Am J Pathol. 2010;176:34–9.
113. Guo T, Zhang L, Chang NE, Singer S, Maki RG, Antonescu CR. Consistent MYC and FLT4 gene amplification in radiation-induced angiosarcoma but not in other radiation-associated atypical vascular lesions. Genes Chromosomes Cancer. 2011;50:25–33. PMID: 20949568.
114. Italiano A, Thomas R, Breen M, Zhang L, Crago AM, Singer S, Khanin R, Maki RG, Mihailovic A, Hafner M, Tuschl T, Antonescu CR. The miR-17-92 cluster and its target THBS1 are differentially expressed in angiosarcomas dependent on MYC amplification. Genes Chromosomes Cancer. 2012;51:569–78. PMID:22383169.
115. Popper H, Thomas L, Telles NC, et al. Development of hepatic angiosarcoma in man induced by vinyl chloride, thorotrast, and arsenic. Am J Pathol. 1978;92:349.
116. Jennings TA, Peterson L, Axiotis CA, et al. Angiosarcoma associated with foreign body material. A report of three cases. Cancer. 1988;62:2436–44.
117. Bessis D, Sotto A, Roubert P, et al. Endothelin-secreting angiosarcoma occurring at the site of an arteriovenous fistula for haemodialysis in a renal transplant recipient. Br J Dermatol. 1998;138:361–3.
118. Leake J, Sheehan MP, Rampling D, et al. Angiosarcoma complicating xeroderma pigmentosum. Histopathology. 1992;21:179–81.
119. Ulbright TM, Clark SA, Einhorn LH. Angiosarcoma associated with germ cell tumors. Hum Pathol. 1985;16:268.
120. Tso CY, Sommer A, Hamoudi AB. Aicardi syndrome, metastatic angiosarcoma of the leg, and scalp lipoma. Am J Med Genet. 1993;45:594.
121. Cafiero F, Gipponi M, Peressini A, et al. Radiation-associated angiosarcoma: diagnostic and therapeutic implications: two case reports and review of the literature. Cancer. 1196;77:249.
122. McLaughlin ER, Brown LF, Weiss SW, et al. VEGF receptors are expressed in a pediatric angiosarcoma in a patient with Aicardi's syndrome. J Invest Dermatol. 2000;114:1209.
123. Cancellieri A, Eusebi V, Mambelli V, et al. Well-differentiated angiosarcoma of the skin following radiotherapy. Report of two cases. Pathol Res Pract. 1991;187:301–6.
124. Caldwell JB, Ryan MT, Benson PM, et al. Cutaneous angiosarcoma arising in the radiation site of a congenital hemangioma. J Am Acad Dermatol. 1995;33:865–70.

125. Lezama-del Valle P, Gerald WL, Tsai J, et al. Malignant vascular tumors in young patients. Cancer. 1998;83:1634–9.
126. Rossi S, Fletcher CD. Angiosarcoma arising in hemangioma/vascular malformation: report of four cases and review of the literature. Am J Sur Pathol. 2002;26:1319.
127. Nord KM, Kandel J, Lefkowitch JH, Lobritto SJ, Morel KD, North PE, Garzon MC. Multiple cutaneous infantile hemangiomas associated with hepatic angiosarcoma: case report and review of the literature. Pediatrics. 2006;118:e907–13. PMID: 16880251.
128. Stewart FW, Treves N. Lymphangiosarcoma in postmastectomy lymphedema. Cancer. 1948; 1:64–81.
129. Folpe AL, Veikkola T, Valtola R, Weiss SW. Vascular endothelial growth factor receptor-3 (VEGFR-3): a marker of vascular tumors with presumed lymphatic differentiation, including Kaposi's sarcoma, kaposiform and Dabska-type hemangioendotheliomas, and a subset of angiosarcomas. Mod Pathol. 2000;13:180–5.
130. Shirley MD, Tang H, Gallione CJ, Baugher JD, Frelin LP, Cohen B, North PE, Marchuk DA, Comi AM, Pevsner J. Sturge-Weber syndrome and port-wine stains caused by somatic mutation in GNAQ. N Engl J Med. 2013;368:1971–9.
131. Sudarsanam A, Ardern-Holmes SL. Sturge-Weber syndrome: from the past to the present. Eur J Paediatr Neurol. 2014;18:257–66.
132. Eerola I, Boon LM, Mulliken JB, Burrows PE, Dompmartin A, Watanabe S, Vanwijck R, Vikkula M. Capillary malformation-arteriovenous malformation, a new clinical and genetic disorder caused by RASA1 mutations. Am J Hum Genet. 2003;73:1240–9. PMID: 14639529.
133. Piccione M, Fragapane T, Antona V, Giachino D, Cupido F, Corsello G. PTEN hamartoma tumor syndromes in childhood: description of two cases and a proposal for follow-up protocol. Am J Med Genet A. 2013;161A(11):2902–8.
134. Luks VL, Kamitaki N, Vivero MP, Uller W, Rab R, Bovée JV, Rialon KL, Guevara CJ, Alomari AI, Greene AK, Fishman SJ, Kozakewich HP, Maclellan RA, Mulliken JB, Rahbar R, Spencer SA, Trenor 3rd CC, Upton J, Zurakowski D, Perkins JA, Kirsh A, Bennett JT, Dobyns WB, Kurek KC, Warman ML, McCarroll SA, Murillo R. Lymphatic and other vascular malformative/overgrowth disorders are caused by somatic mutations in PIK3CA. J Pediatr. 2015;166(4):1048–54. PMID: 25681199.
135. Lee MS, Liang MG, Mulliken JB. Diffuse capillary malformation with overgrowth: a clinical subtype of vascular anomalies with hypertrophy. J Am Acad Dermatol. 2013;69(4):589–94. PMID: 23906555.
136. Couto JA, Huang L, Vivero MP, Kamitaki N, Maclellan RA, Mulliken JB, Bischoff J, Warman ML, Greene AK. Abstract 72: endothelial cells from capillary malformations are enriched for somatic GNAQ mutations and aberrantly express PDGFRβ. Plastic Reconstr Surg. 2015;135:56.
137. Comi AM. Update on Sturge-Weber syndrome: diagnosis, treatment, quantitative measures, and controversies. Lymphat Res Biol. 2007;5:257–64.
138. Piram M, Lorette G, Sirinelli D, Herbreteau D, Giraudeau B, Maruani A. Sturge-Weber syndrome in patients with facial port-wine stain. Pediatr Dermatol. 2012;29:32–7.
139. Ch'ng S, Tan ST. Facial port-wine stains – clinical stratification and risks of neuro-ocular involvement. J Plast Reconstr Aesthet Surg. 2008;61:889–93.
140. North PE, Sanchez-Carpintero I, Mizeracki A, Waner M, Mihm MC. The distinctive histology of lip enlargement in port-wine stains: a clinicopathological study. Lab Invest. 2003;83(1):96A.
141. Sanchez-Carpintero I, Mihm MC, Waner M, Mizeracki A, North PE. Epithelial and mesenchymal hamartomatous changes in mature port-wine stains: morphological evidence for a multiple germ layer field defect. J Am Acad Dermatol. 2004;50(4):606–12.
142. Finley JL, Clark RA, Colvin RB, et al. Immunofluorescent staining with antibodies to factor VIII, fibronectin, and collagenous basement membrane protein in normal human skin and port wine stains. Arch Dermatol. 1982;118:971–5.
143. Barsky SH, Rosen S, Geer DE, Noe JM. The nature and evolution of port wine stains: a computer-assisted study. J Invest Dermatol. 1980;74:154–7.
144. Smoller BR, Rosen S. Port-wine stains. A disease of altered neural modulation of blood vessels? Arch Dermatol. 1986;122:177–9.

145. Rydh M, Malm M, Jernbeck J, et al. Ectatic blood vessels in port-wine stains lack innervation: possible role in pathogenesis. Plast Reconstr Surg. 1991;87:419–22.
146. Weinstein LS, Shenker A, Gejman PV, Merino MJ, Friedman E, Spiegel AM. Activating mutations of the stimulatory G protein in the McCune–Albright syndrome. N Engl J Med. 1991;325:1688–95. PubMed: 1944469.
147. Van Raamsdonk CD, Bezrookove V, Green G, et al. Frequent somatic mutations of GNAQ in uveal melanoma and blue naevi. Nature. 2009;457:599–602. PubMed: 19078957.
148. Calvert JT, Riney TJ, Kontos CD, et al. Allelic and locus heterogeneity in inherited venous malformations. Hum Mol Genet. 1999;8:1279–89.
149. Vikkula M, Boon LM, Carraway KL, 3rd, et al. Vascular dysmorphogenesis caused by an activating mutation in the receptor tyrosine kinase TIE2. [see comments]. Cell. 1996;87:1181–90.
150. Limaye N, Wouters V, Uebelhoer M, Tuominen M, Wirkkala R, et al. Somatic mutations in angiopoietin receptor gene TEK cause solitary and multiple sporadic venous malformations. Nat Genet. 2009;41:118–24.
151. Wouters V, et al. Hereditary cutaneomucosal venous malformations are caused by TIE2 mutations with widely variable hyper-phosphorylating effects. Eur J Hum Genet. 2010;18:414–20.
152. Soblet J, Limaye N, Uebelhoer M, Boon LM, Vikkula M. Variable somatic TIE2 mutations in half of sporadic venous malformations. Mol Syndromol. 2013;4:179–83.
153. Uebelhoer M, et al. Venous malformation-causative TIE2 mutations mediate an AKT-dependent decrease in PDGFB. Hum Mol Genet. 2013;22:3438–48.
154. Bean WB. Anomylous vascular spiders and related lesions of the skin. Springfield: Charles C. Thomas; 1958.
155. Nguyen H-L, Boon LM, Vikkula M. Genetics of vascular malformations. Semin Pediatr Surg. 2014;23:221–6.
156. Imperial R, Helwig EB. Verrucous hemangioma. A clinicopathologic study of 21 cases. Arch Dermatol. 1967;96(3):247–53. PMID: 6038751.
157. Mankani MH, Dufresne CR. Verrucous malformations: their presentation and management. Ann Plast Surg. 2000;45:31–6.
158. Mulliken JB. Capillary malformations, hyperkeratotic stains, and miscellaneous vascular blots. In: Mulliken & Young's vascular anomalies: hemangiomas and malformations, 2nd edn. Oxford: Oxford University Press; 2013, p. 538.
159. Couto JA, Vivero MP, Kozakewich HP, Taghinia AH, Mulliken JB, Warman ML, Greene AK. A somatic MAP3K3 mutation is associated with verrucous venous malformation. Am J Hum Genet. 2015;96:480–6. PMID: 25728774.
160. Tennant LB, Mulliken JB, Perez-Atayde AR, Kozakewich HP. Verrucous hemangioma revisited. Pediatr Dermatol. 2006;23:208–15.
161. Wang L, Gao T, Wang G. Verrucous hemangioma: a clinicopathological and immunohistochemical analysis of 74 cases. J Cutan Pathol. 2014;41:823–30.
162. Laing EL, Brasch HD, Steel R, Jia J, Itinteang T, Tan ST, Day DJ. Verrucous hemangioma expresses primitive markers. J Cutan Pathol. 2013;40:391–6.
163. Mounayer C, Wassef M, Enjolras O, et al. Facial 'glomangiomas': large facial venous malformations with glomus cells. J Am Acad Dermatol. 2001;45:239–45.
164. Gould EW, Manivel JC, Albores-Saavedra J, et al. Locally infiltrative glomus tumors and glomangiosarcomas. A clinical, ultrastructural, and immunohistochemical study. Cancer. 1990;65:310–8.
165. Yang JS, Ko JW, Suh KS, et al. Congenital multiple plaque-like glomangiomyoma. Am J Dermatopathol. 1999;21:454–7.
166. Rycroft RJ, Menter MA, Sharvill DE, et al. Hereditary multiple glomus tumours. Report of four families and a review of literature. Trans St Johns Hosp Dermatol Soc. 1975;61:70–81.
167. Wood WS, Dimmick JE. Multiple infiltrating glomus tumors in children. Cancer. 1977;40:1680–5.
168. Boon LM, Mulliken JB, Enjolras O, et al. Glomulovenous malformation (glomangioma) and venous malformation: distinct clinicopathologic and genetic entities. Arch Dermatol. 2004; 140:971–6.

169. Irrthum A, Brouillard P, Enjolras O, et al. Linkage disequilibrium narrows locus for venous malformation with glomus cells (VMGLOM) to a single 1.48 Mbp YAC. Eur J Hum Genet. 2001;9:34–8.
170. Brouillard P, Olsen BR, Vikkula M. High-resolution physical and transcript map of the locus for venous malformations with glomus cells (VMGLOM) on chromosome 1p21-p22. Genomics. 2000;67:96–101.
171. Brouillard P, Boon LM, Vikkula M. Mutations in a novel factor, glomulin, are responsible for glomuvenous malformations ("glomangiomas"). Am J Hum Genet. 2002;70:866–74.
172. Brouillard P, Boon LM, Revencu N, Berg J, Dompmartin A, Dubois J, Garzon M, Holden S, Kangesu L, Labrèze C, Lynch SA, McKeown C, Meskauskas R, Quere I, Syed S, Vabres P, Wassef M, Mulliken JB, Vikkula M, GVM Study Group. Genotypes and phenotypes of 162 families with a glomulin mutation. Mol Syndromol. 2013;4:157–64.
173. Amyere M, Aerts V, Brouillard P, McIntyre BA, Duhoux FP, Wassef M, Enjolras O, Mulliken JB, Devuyst O, Antoine-Poirel H, Boon LM, Vikkula M. Somatic uniparental isodisomy explains multifocality of glomuvenous malformations. Am J Hum Genet. 2013;92:188–96.
174. Grisendi S, Chambraud B, Gout I, Comoglio PM, Crepaldi T. Ligand-regulated binding of FAP68 to the hepatocyte growth factor receptor. J Biol Chem. 2001;276:46632–8.
175. Chambraud B, Radanyi C, Camonis JH, Shazand K, Rajkowski K, Baulieu E. FAP48, a new protein that forms specific complexes with both immunophilins FKBP59 and FKBP12: prevention by the immunosuppressant drugs FK506 and rapamycin. J Biol Chem. 1996;271:32923–9.
176. Tron AE, Arai T, Duda DM, Kuwabara H, Olszewski JL, Fujiwara Y, Bahamon BN, Signoretti S, Schulman BA, DeCaprio JA. The glomuvenous malformation protein glomulin binds Rbx1 and regulates cullin RING ligase-mediated turnover of Fbw7. Mol Cell. 2012;46:67–78.
177. McIntyre BA, Brouillard P, Aerts V, Gutierrez-Roelens I, Vikkula M. Glomulin is predominantly expressed in vascular smooth muscle cells in the embryonic and adult mouse. Gene Expr Patterns. 2004;4:351–8.
178. Enjolras O, Logeart I, Gelbert F, et al. Arteriovenous malformations: a study of 200 cases. Ann Dermatol Venereol (Fr). 1999;127:17–22.
179. Bluefarb SM, Adams LA. Arteriovenous malformation with angiodermatitis. Stasis dermatitis simulating Kaposi's disease. Arch Dermatol. 1967;96:176–81. PMID: 6039154.
180. Guttmacher AE, Marchuk DA, White RI. Hereditary hemorrhagic telangiectasia. N Engl J Med. 1995;333:918–24.
181. Abdalla SA, Letarte M. Hereditary haemorrhagic telangiectasia: current views on genetics and mechanisms of disease. J Med Genet. 2006;43:97–110.
182. Revencu N, Boon LM, Mendola A, et al. RASA1 mutations and associated phenotypes in 68 families with capillary malformation-arteriovenous malformation. Hum Mutat. 2013;34:1632–41.
183. Kim C, Ko CJ, Baker KE, Antaya RJ. Histopathologic and ultrasound characteristics of cutaneous capillary malformations in a patient with capillary malformation-arteriovenous malformation syndrome. Pediatr Dermatol. 2015;32:128–31.
184. Kozakewich HPW, Mulliken JB. Histopathology of vascular malformations. In: Mulliken & Young's vascular anomalies: hemangiomas and malformations, 2nd edn. Oxford: Oxford University Press; 2013. p. 500–1.
185. Kozakewich HPW, Mulliken JB. Histopathology of vascular malformations. In: Mulliken & Young's vascular anomalies: hemangiomas and malformations, 2nd edn. Oxford: Oxford University Press; 2013. p. 488.
186. Hershkovitz D, Bercovich D, Sprecher E, Lapidot M. RASA1 mutations may cause hereditary capillary malformations without arteriovenous malformations. Br J Dermatol. 2008;158: 1035–40.
187. Thiex R, Mulliken JB, Revencu N, Boon LM, Burrows PE, Cordisco M, Dwight Y, Smith ER, Vikkula M, Orbach DB. A novel association between RASA1 mutations and spinal arteriovenous anomalies. Am J Neuroradiol. 2010;31:775–9.
188. Wooderchak-Donahue W, Stevenson DA, McDonald J, Grimmer JF, Gedge F, Bayrak-Toydemir P. RASA1 analysis: clinical and molecular findings in a series of consecutive cases. Eur J Med Genet. 2012;55:91–5.

189. Henkemeyer M, Rossi DJ, Holmyard DP, Puri MC, Mbamalu G, Harpal K, Shih TS, Jacks T, Pawson T. Vascular system defects and neuronal apoptosis in mice lacking ras GTPase-activating protein. Nature. 1995;377:695–701.
190. Friedman E, Gejman PV, Martin GA, McCormick F. Nonsense mutations in the C-terminal SH2 region of the GTPase activating protein (GAP) gene in human tumours. Nat Genet. 1993;5:242–7.
191. Burrows PE, Gonzalez-Garay ML, Rasmussen JC, Aldrich MB, Guilliod R, Maus EA, Fife CE, Kwon S, Lapinski PE, King PD, Sevick-Muraca EM. Lymphatic abnormalities are associated with RASA1 gene mutations in mouse and man. Proc Natl Acad Sci U S A. 2013;110: 8621–6.
192. Lubeck BA, Lapinski PE, Bauler TJ, Oliver JA, Hughes ED, Saunders TL, King PD. Blood vascular abnormalities in Rasa1(R780Q) knockin mice: implications for the pathogenesis of capillary malformation-arteriovenous malformation. Am J Pathol. 2014;184:3163–9.
193. Lapinski PE, Kwon S, Lubeck BA, Wilkinson JE, Srinivasan RS, Sevick-Muraca E, King PD. RASA1 maintains the lymphatic vasculature in a quiescent functional state in mice. J Clin Invest. 2012;122:733–47.
194. Kawasaki J, Aegerter S, Fevurly RD, Mammoto A, Mammoto T, Sahin M, Mably JD, Fishman SJ, Chan J. RASA1 functions in EPHB4 signaling pathway to suppress endothelial mTORC1 activity. J Clin Invest. 2014;124:2774–84.
195. McAllister KA, Grogg KM, Johnson DW, et al. Endoglin, a TGF-beta binding protein of endothelial cells, is the gene for hereditary haemorrhagic telangiectasia type 1. Nat Genet. 1994;8:345–51.
196. Johnson DW, Berg JN, Baldwin MA, et al. Mutations in the activin receptor-like kinase 1 gene in hereditary haemorrhagic telangiectasia type 2. Nat Genet. 1996;13:189–95.
197. Gallione CJ, Repetto GM, Legius E, et al. A combined syndrome of juvenile polyposis and hereditary haemorrhagic telangiectasia associated with mutations in MADH4 32. (SMAD4). Lancet. 2004;363(9412):852–9.
198. Tillet E, Bailly S. Emerging roles of BMP9 and BMP10 in hereditary hemorrhagic telangiectasia. Front Genet. 2015;8;5:456.
199. Wooderchak-Donahue WL, McDonald J, O'Fallon B, Upton PD, Li W, Roman BL, Young S, Plant P, Fülöp GT, Langa C, Morrell NW, Botella LM, Bernabeu C, Stevenson DA, Runo JR, Bayrak-Toydemir P. BMP9 mutations cause a vascular-anomaly syndrome with phenotypic overlap with hereditary hemorrhagic telangiectasia. Am J Hum Genet. 2013;5; 93:530–7.
200. Sansal I, Sellers WR. The biology and clinical relevance of the PTEN tumor suppressor pathway. J Clin Oncol. 2004;22:2954–63.
201. Brewis C, Pracy JP, Albert DM. Treatment of lymphangiomas of the head and neck in children by intralesional injection of OK-432 (Picibanil). Clin Otolaryngol. 2000;25:130–5.
202. Molitch HI, Unger EC, White EL, et al. Percutaneous sclerotherapy of lymphangiomas. Radiology. 1995;194:343–7. Lancet. 2004;363:852–9.
203. Easterly NB. Cutaneous hemangiomas, vascular stains and malformations, and associated syndromes [Review]. Probl Dermatol. 1995;7:67–108.
204. Chitayat D, Kalousek DK, Bamforth JS, et al. Lymphatic abnormalities in fetuses with posterior cervical cystic hydroma. Am J Med Genet. 1989;33:352–6.
205. Kurek KC, Luks VL, Ayturk UM, Alomari AI, Fishman SJ, Spenser SA, et al. Somatic activating mutations in PIK3CA cause CLOVES syndrome. Am J Hum Genet. 2012;90:1108–15.
206. Lee JH, Huynh M, Silhavy JL, Kim S, Dixon-Salazar T, Heiberg A, et al. De novo somatic mutations in components of the PI3K-AKT3-mTOR pathway cause hemimegalencephaly. Nat Genet. 2012;44:941–5.
207. Maclellan RA, Luks VL, Vivero MP, Mulliken JB, Zurakowski D, Padwa BL, et al. PIK3CA activating mutations in facial infiltrating lipomatosis. Plast Reconstr Surg. 2014;133:12e–9.
208. Samuels Y, Wang Z, Bardelli A, Silliman N, Ptak J, Szabo S, et al. High frequency of mutations of the PIK3CA gene in human cancers. Science. 2004;304:554.
209. Kinross KM, Montgomery KG, Kleinschmidt M, Waring P, Ivetac I, Tikoo A, et al. An activating Pik3ca mutation coupled with Pten loss is sufficient to initiate ovarian tumorigenesis in mice. J Clin Invest. 2012;122:553–7.

Chapter 2
Vascular Overgrowth

Kelly J. Duffy, Michael E. Kelly, and David Bick

Blood and lymphatic vessel formation is a vital dynamic process that when dysregulated can lead to excessive or abnormal formation of the vasculature. Vascular malformations are often associated with bony and/or soft tissue hypertrophy (overgrowth) that may occur regionally or involve the whole body. These overgrowth syndromes can be categorized based on the type of vascular malformation present (Table 2.1). The purpose of this review is to provide an overview of the features, pathogenesis, and molecular mechanisms involved in overgrowth syndromes associated with vascular malformations.

Overgrowth Syndromes Associated with Slow-Flow Vascular Malformations

Congenital Lipomatous Asymmetric Overgrowth, Vascular Malformation, Epidermal Nevus, and Skeletal Anomalies (CLOVES) Syndrome

CLOVES syndrome is a sporadic disorder characterized by truncal lipomatous masses, vascular malformations, and cutaneous and acral/musculoskeletal anomalies [1, 2]. Its delineation came from a group of patients with overlapping clinical

K.J. Duffy, PhD (✉)
Department of Radiology, Medical College of Wisconsin, Milwaukee, WI, USA
e-mail: kjduffy10@gmail.com

M.E. Kelly, MD, PhD
Pediatrics Department, Division of Pediatric Hematology, Oncology, Bone Marrow Transplantation, Children's Hospital of Wisconsin, Milwaukee, WI, USA

D. Bick, MD
Pediatrics Department, Medical College of Wisconsin, Milwaukee, WI, USA

© Springer Science+Business Media New York 2016
P.E. North, T. Sander (eds.), *Vascular Tumors and Developmental Malformations*,
Molecular and Translational Medicine, DOI 10.1007/978-1-4939-3240-5_2

Table 2.1 Syndromes associated with vascular malformations

Syndromes associated with slow-flow lesions	Syndromes associated with fast-flow lesions
Klippel-Trenaunay syndrome (KTS)	PTEN hamartoma tumor syndromes (PHTS) • Cowden syndrome • Bannayan-Riley-Ruvalcaba syndrome (BRRS) • SOLAMEN syndrome
Cutis marmorata telangiectatica congenita (CMTC)	Capillary malformation-arteriovenous malformation (CM-AVM) syndrome
Megalencephaly-capillary malformation (MCAP) Macrocephaly-capillary malformation (M-CM) syndrome	Parkes Weber syndrome (PKWS)
CLOVES syndrome	
Proteus syndrome	
Beckwith-Wiedemann syndrome	

characteristics who did not meet the specific diagnostic criteria for Proteus syndrome (Table 2.2). The dysregulated adipose tissue, scoliosis, and enlarged bony structures in CLOVES are not progressive or structurally distorting like those seen in Proteus syndrome [1], and the overgrowth in CLOVES syndrome is congenital, "ballooning" in nature, grows proportionately with the patient, and often affects both feet [1, 3].

In 2012, Kurek and colleagues reported their finding of activating mutations in *PIK3CA* as the cause of CLOVES syndrome [4]. This group used massively parallel sequencing of DNA or RNA recovered from affected tissue from individuals with CLOVES syndrome who had undergone surgical resection of lipomatous overgrowth or vascular malformation with lipomatous overgrowth. Mutations were not detected in blood or saliva DNA from individuals who had mutations in their affected tissue. This supports Happle's theory of paradominant inheritance of a single gene to explain the occurrence of both familial and sporadic cases [5–7]. This could occur if individuals heterozygous for a defective gene were phenotypically normal, and only those with a somatic mutation resulting in loss of heterozygosity of the gene would develop the syndrome. Such a mechanism would result in a clonal population of cells homozygous or hemizygous for the mutation and could explain the mosaic pattern of lesions in KTS (Fig. 2.1). Happle suggests that homozygous expression of the genetic defect would likely be incompatible with life [7], which would explain the sporadic and apparent non-Mendelian inheritance pattern. Interestingly, the *PIK3CA* mutations discovered in CLOVES syndrome have been detected in several types of cancer [8]. This finding also underscores the importance of the PI3K-AKT pathway (Fig. 2.2) in overgrowth syndromes known to result from related activating mutations (Table 2.1).

Table 2.2 Diagnostic criteria for Proteus syndrome

Diagnostic criteria for Proteus syndrome	
For diagnosis: *general criteria* (*mandatory*)	*Specific criteria* (*category signs*)
Mosaic distribution of lesions	Either one from A or
Progressive course	Two from B or
Sporadic occurrence	Three from C
Category signs	Manifestations
A.	1. Connective tissue nevus
B.	1. Epidermal nevus

	2. Disproportionate overgrowth (one or more)
	   Limbs
	      Arms/legs
	      Hands/feet/digits
	   Skull
	      Hyperostoses
	   External auditory meatus
	      Hyperostosis
	   Vertebrae
	      Megaspondylodysplasia
	   Viscera
	      Spleen/thymus

	3. Specific tumors before end of second decade
	   Bilateral ovarian cystadenomas
	   Parotid monomorphic adenoma

C.	1. Dysregulated adipose tissue (either one)
	   Lipomas
	   Regional absence of fat

	2. Vascular malformations (one or more)
	   Capillary malformation
	   Venous malformation
	   Lymphatic malformation

	3. Facial phenotype
	   Dolichocephaly
	   Long face
	   Minor downslanting of palpebral fissures
	   and/or minor ptosis
	   Low nasal bridge
	   Wide or anteverted nares
	   Open mouth at rest

Adapted from Biesecker et al. [9]

Proteus Syndrome

Proteus syndrome is a rare sporadic disorder characterized by soft tissue and bony hypertrophy of the hands and feet, hemihypertrophy, cranial hyperostosis, dysregulated adipose tissue, vascular malformations, and connective tissue and epidermal nevi. There are strict diagnostic criteria for Proteus syndrome, listed in Table 2.2

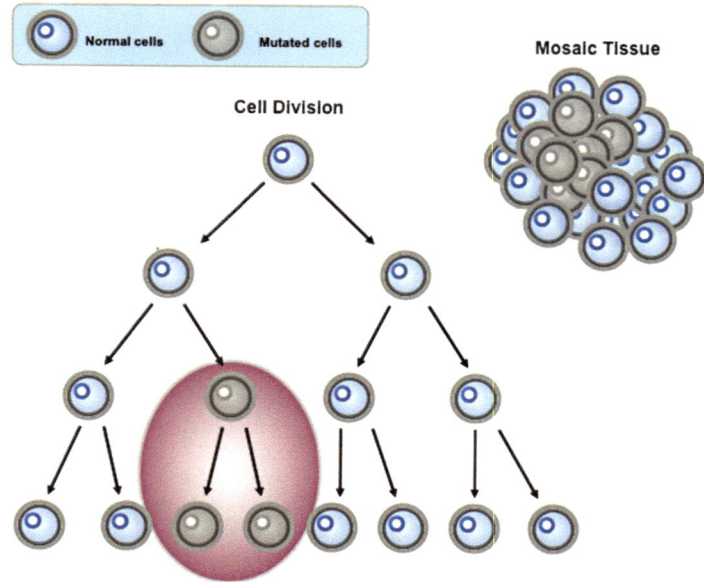

Fig. 2.1 *Representation of somatic mosaicism.* Mosaic distribution of lesions in vascular anomalies and associated overgrowth syndromes is postulated to occur via a post-zygotic mutation resulting in a subpopulation of cells with the mutation among a population of normal cells with no mutation

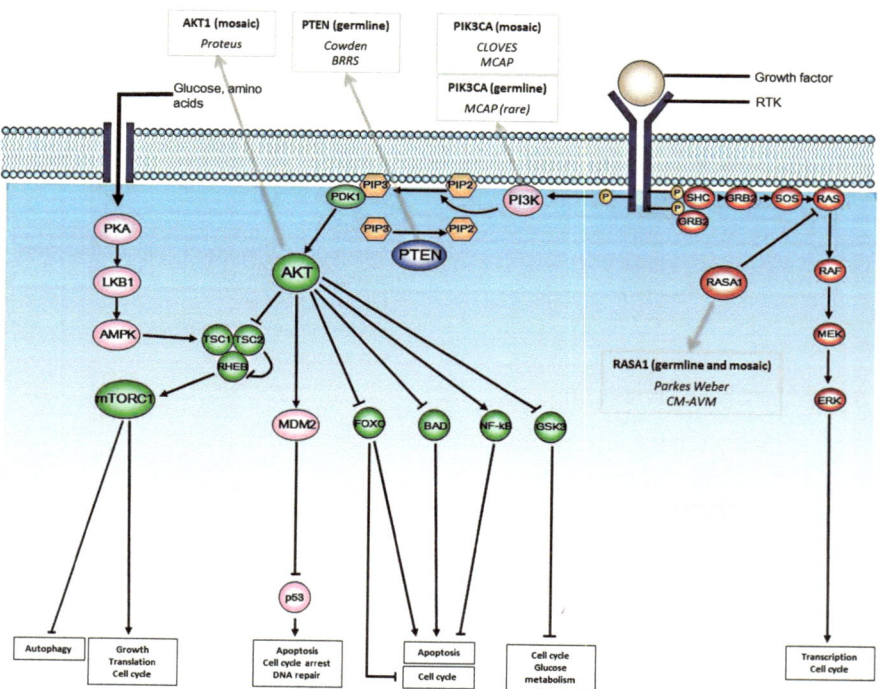

Fig. 2.2 Schematic of the PI3K/AKT pathway

[9]. Diagnosed patients are required to meet both general and specific criteria, with the general characteristics of mosaic distribution of lesions, progressive clinical course, and sporadic occurrence mandatory criteria. The vascular malformations associated with Proteus syndrome are not well characterized, although clinical observation suggests that slow-flow lesions (capillary, venous, and lymphatic malformations) similar to KTS may occur.

In 2011, Lindhurst et al. found a mosaic activating mutation in *AKT1* associated with Proteus syndrome [10]. The p.Glu17Lys mutations were detected in affected lesion tissue, but not in unaffected tissue samples from the same individual. Like CLOVES syndrome, this finding supports Happle's original hypothesis of somatic mosaicism that is lethal in the non-mosaic state [5, 6]. This idea is substantiated by the mosaic pattern of lesions in Proteus syndrome as well as the report of discordance in identical twin pairs [1].

Klippel-Trenaunay Syndrome (KTS)

KTS is characterized by regional overgrowth of soft tissue and bony structures with associated superficial capillary malformations, varicose veins, and/or venous malformations. Lymphatic malformations occur in about 11 % of patients [11]. The cutaneous capillary stain and venous malformations are often noted at birth and are associated with limb hypertrophy. Involvement of lower extremities is typical; however, 10–15 % of cases involve both the upper and lower extremities [12]. Affected limbs are commonly longer with an increased circumference when compared with the unaffected limb. The limb length discrepancy may be slight or dramatic and may become prominent with age, though progression is unpredictable. Limb enlargement tends to slow or stop once the child's growth cycle is complete [11]. Macrodactyly, syndactyly, and hypertrophy of the thorax, pelvis, abdomen, head, or neck can also occur [13].

On histological exam, the capillary malformations (CMs) in KTS consist of an increased number of abnormal ectatic capillaries with flat endothelial cells (ECs) in the papillary dermis [14]. The lymphatic malformations typically accompanying the CMs display dilated lymphatic vessels filled with lymph fluid [14], whereas the venous malformations can include aneurismal dilation, aplasia, hypoplasia, duplication, or anomalous vessels [13].

The origin of KTS is unknown, and most cases are sporadic in nature. However, Aelvoet, Jorens, and Roelen reported familial cases of KTS suggesting a multifactorial pattern of inheritance [15]. Additionally, there have been reports of de novo chromosomal abnormalities in three different KTS patients [16–18], although no candidate genes have been verified in larger KTS populations. These reports suggest that genetic factors may contribute to the development and pathogenesis of KTS. Given the overlapping clinical characteristics between KTS and other overgrowth syndromes such as CLOVES syndrome and Proteus syndrome, it is possible that KTS also results from mutations in components of the PI3K-AKT pathway. To date, no such mutations have been reported.

Cutis Marmorata Telangiectatica Congenita (CMTC)

CMTC is a low-flow vascular malformation characterized by a fixed coarsely reticulated vascular pattern on the skin that is usually noted at birth and can have a localized or generalized distribution. CMTC is associated with congenital anomalies in 27–50 % of cases [19, 20]. These anomalies are more often found in generalized cases of CMTC. The most frequent anomaly is limb hypoplasia [12]. However, other growth abnormalities can also be associated with CMTC such as limb hypertrophy, skull asymmetry, and syndactyly [19–22].

Histologic studies have been inconsistent with some studies reporting dilated capillaries in the dermis and subcutaneous tissue, while others were unable to detect a vascular anomaly [12]. Picascia and Esterly reported sparse dermal perivascular lymphocytic infiltrates and swelling of endothelial cells [19]. The cause of CMTC is unknown, and it appears to occur sporadically. Several theories have been presented to explain this disorder. One case series suggested a common dysmorphogenic environmental agent in the pathogenesis [23], while others propose genetic mosaicism in which the lethal gene survives via partial or mosaic expression [24, 25]. Once again, Happle's theory of paradominant inheritance has also been proposed for CMTC [26].

Megalencephaly-Capillary Malformation (MCAP)

MCAP, previously known as Macrocephaly-Capillary Malformation (M-CM) syndrome, is a rare sporadic disorder distinct from cutis marmorata telangiectatica congenita (CMTC), although the vascular pattern can appear similar. MCAP syndrome is characterized by a CMTC-like vascular malformation in association with macrocephaly and developmental delay. While MCAP syndrome resembles the vascular malformation in CMTC, the skin lesion in MCAP syndrome is a reticulated capillary malformation rather than a true CMTC, as there is no ulceration or cutaneous atrophy associated with the lesion [27]. Often, a midline facial capillary malformation is reported, with other associations including hydrocephalus, connective tissue defects, toe syndactyly, frontal bossing, and hemihypertrophy [27, 28].

Recently, Riviere and colleagues discovered de novo germline and post-zygotic mutations in *PIK3CA* associated with MCAP [29]. These mutations, like those found in *PIK3CA* in Proteus syndrome, are activating mutations that result in elevated PI3K-AKT pathway activity (Fig. 2.2) [29].

Beckwith-Wiedemann Syndrome

Beckwith-Wiedemann is a syndrome characterized primarily by gigantism, macroglossia, and omphalocele [30], but may also include posterior helical ear pits, hypoglycemia, a predisposition to tumors, and facial capillary malformations. The capillary malformations are usually centrofacial and virtually identical to, but more persistent than, salmon patches (nevus simplex).

Most cases of Beckwith-Wiedemann syndrome are sporadic, but there have also been reports of autosomal dominant inheritance within families. Cytogenetic analysis has demonstrated dysregulation of a region on chromosome 11p15 composed of two distinct domains of imprinted genes regulated by two imprinting centers [31, 32]. (Epi)genomic alterations in this region have been associated with approximately 80 % of Beckwith-Wiedemann cases [33]. Within these domains, overexpression of key imprinted genes has been identified to contribute to disease pathogenesis, IGF2 and H19 in domain 1 and LIT-1 and p57^{KIP2} in domain 2. The molecular alterations in domain 1 only occur in 5 % of Beckwith-Wiedemann patients, whereas imprinting defects within domain 2 account for roughly 50 % of molecular defects in affected individuals [33]. Rare mutations have been identified in families with autosomal dominant inheritance and primarily involve the p57^{KIP2} gene. It has been suggested that p57^{KIP2} mutations are related to embryonal tumor types like rhabdomyosarcoma and hepatoblastoma, whereas upregulation of IGF2 has been more commonly associated with Wilms' tumor [32]. Paternal uniparental disomy (UPD) involving both domain 1 and domain 2 is found in approximately 20 % of Beckwith-Wiedemann cases [33]. Given that these individuals with UPD exhibit somatic mosaicism of lesions, it is possible that this molecular defect is caused by a post-zygotic event [33].

Overgrowth Syndromes Associated with High-Flow Vascular Malformations

PTEN Hamartoma Tumor Syndromes (PHTS)

The PHTS is a spectrum of autosomal dominant hamartomatous disorders with phenotypic variability caused by germline mutations of the tumor suppressor gene phosphatase and tensin homolog deleted on chromosome 10 (PTEN) [34–40]. Cowden syndrome (CS) and Bannayan-Riley-Ruvalcaba syndrome (BRRS) are the most commonly reported syndromes within the PHTS spectrum [34–40]. A variety of vascular malformations have been reported in patients with BRRS or CS [41, 42]. These lesions are most frequently deep vascular anomalies that are almost all fast-flow with unusual characteristics including multifocal distribution, musculoskeletal location, ectopic adipose tissue, and drainage into dilated veins [43]. In addition to vascular anomalies, both BRRS and CS are also characterized by lipomatosis, macrocephaly, and hamartomatous lesions involving the skin, mucous membranes, GI tract, thyroid, breast, brain, and genitourinary system. A more recently described syndrome classified as part of the PHTS spectrum is the segmental overgrowth, lipomatosis, arteriovenous malformation, and epidermal nevus (SOLAMEN) syndrome [44] This syndrome is distinct from CS and BRRS as it involves complex congenital dysmorphisms including segmental overgrowth and epidermal nevi in addition to the other associated phenotypes. While similar to Proteus syndrome, individuals with SOLAMEN syndrome do not meet the strict diagnostic criteria for Proteus [9, 44].

The PHTS disorders are associated with germline mutations in the tumor suppressor gene PTEN. Although CS and BRRS are often differentiated by clinical characteristics, investigations have been unable to determine specific genotype-phenotype correlations. A single mutation in PTEN has resulted in both CS and BRRS within a family [45]. This suggests that CS and BRRS actually represent one condition with a phenotype continuum that could be influenced by host factors or additional somatic mutations. It has been shown that SOLAMEN syndrome is also associated with a germline mutation in PTEN; however, analysis of lesional tissues demonstrated a second molecular event at the PTEN locus resulting in deletion of the remaining wild-type allele [44].

Capillary Malformation-Arteriovenous Malformation (CM-AVM)

CM-AVM is a hereditary disorder characterized by multifocal cutaneous capillary malformations in association with high-flow vascular malformations, such as AVMs or arteriovenous fistulas (AVFs). These high-flow lesions are often found in the skin, subcutaneous tissue, bone, muscle, and brain. The capillary malformations tend to present as small pink to red macules often surrounded by a pale halo and may be widely distributed cutaneously. There have also been reports of larger solitary capillary malformations associated with CM-AVM [46].

CM-AVM is an autosomal dominant disorder caused by loss-of-function mutations in the RASA1 gene [47]. The molecular mechanisms by which these mutations lead to the localized vascular phenotype are unknown, although they likely involve the loss of inhibition of RAS p21 by the RASA1 protein. RAS p21 is a protein that controls cellular growth, proliferation, survival, and differentiation, indicating a potential role in the vascular overgrowth. The variable location within the skin, subcutaneous tissue, bone, muscle, and brain and intrafamilial presentations may suggest a second molecular event (second hit) is necessary.

Parkes Weber Syndrome (PKWS)

Parkes Weber syndrome is the association of high-flow lesions (AVM or AVF) with capillary malformation(s) and overgrowth of the affected extremity. Lymphatic malformations and lymphedema may also be present [12]. It seems that PKWS is a clinically and etiologically heterogeneous disorder, as RASA1 mutations have been found to occur in affected individuals with multifocal capillary malformations but not those with a solitary lesion [48]. Like CM-AVM syndrome, a second-hit mechanism may be involved in affected tissue, although this mechanism has not been demonstrated in PKWS.

Vascular Malformations and Associated Overgrowth: Etiology

Tissue overgrowth results from dysfunction of processes that control apoptosis, cellular proliferation, and cell growth. One signaling pathway that contributes to this regulatory process is the phosphoinositide-3-kinase (PI3K)-AKT pathway (Fig. 2.2). Numerous animal studies provided evidence that disruption of the PI3K/AKT pathway results in disordered growth [49–55]. In addition, advances in the field of vascular anomalies' research have led to the discovery of numerous human diseases of abnormal growth that are associated with defects in the pathway. Some of the first examples in human disease were the PHTS disorders, which result from loss-of-function mutations in the PTEN gene that negatively regulates the PI3K/AKT pathway. PTEN is a dual phosphatase protein that negatively regulates the PI3K/AKT pathway, a pathway essential to cellular growth and survival. When PTEN function is disrupted, the activation of this pathway increases. It is possible that the germline PTEN mutation with a subsequent second hit in somatic tissue could be a result in the various forms of overgrowth seen in PHTS, with the type and extent of overgrowth determined by the timing of the event and the cell type affected. However, this theory has yet to be validated. Additional evidence demonstrating the importance of this pathway came from the identification of RASA1 mutations in CM-AVM syndrome and PKWS. Ras positively regulates signaling of pathways involved in cellular growth and proliferation, including the PI3K/AKT pathway. RASA1 functions through inhibition of Ras, thus loss of RASA1 function results in loss of Ras inhibition and uncontrolled pathway activation.

More recently, activating mutations in *PIK3CA* were found to be associated with Proteus syndrome and MCAP. *PIK3CA* encodes the 110-kD catalytic alpha subunit of PI3K, which is activated upon tyrosine kinase receptor ligand binding. Activated PI3K converts phosphatidylinositol (3,4)-bisphosphate (PIP2) to phosphatidylinositol (3,4,5)-triphosphate (PIP3) and subsequently leads to the translocation and phosphorylation of PDK1, which then phosphorylates AKT. AKT then exerts its downstream effects on PI3K-AKT pathway constituents. This occurs more directly in the case of CLOVES syndrome, as the activating mutations in this syndrome are found in AKT1 [4]. Though mutations in the PI3K-AKT pathway were identified, the mechanisms and understanding related to variable phenotypic presentation in individuals with the same mutation are still unclear. While genetic causes have not yet been delineated for some other overgrowth syndromes, the potential of PI3K-AKT pathway involvement is clear and warrants further investigation.

Overgrowth syndromes associated with vascular malformations represent a spectrum of disorders with variable clinical presentations and molecular associations that are challenging to diagnose, manage, and treat clinically. Although phenotypically heterogeneous, a common characteristic among this spectrum is the mosaic nature of the overgrowth and the presence of more than one affected cell lineage [56]. This suggests that the molecular insult responsible for these syndromes could be explained by Happle's theory of a post-zygotic somatic mutation that is lethal in a germline state [6]. The evidence provided by several groups who identified somatic activating mutations associated with overgrowth syndromes supports Happle's theory, as the somatic changes resulted in altered expression of PI3K pathway components detectable only in the lesion tissue of affected individuals. The variable clinical phenotypes and severity of the lesions are likely to be determined by the timing, location, and nature of the secondary event, though this has not been confirmed [47, 56]. Future studies to investigate this relationship as well as the potential that the PI3K-AKT pathway offers for therapeutic development will likely yield opportunities for intervention in individuals with overgrowth syndromes associated with vascular malformations.

References

1. Sapp JC, Turner JT, van de Kamp JM, van Dijk FS, Lowry RB, Biesecker LG. Newly delineated syndrome of congenital lipomatous overgrowth, vascular malformations, and epidermal nevi (CLOVE syndrome) in seven patients. Am J Med Genet A. 2007;143A(24):2944–58.
2. Alomari AI. Characterization of a distinct syndrome that associates complex truncal overgrowth, vascular, and acral anomalies: a descriptive study of 18 cases of CLOVES syndrome. Clin Dysmorphol. 2009;18(1):1–7.
3. Gucev ZS, Tasic V, Jancevska A, Konstantinova MK, Pop-Jordanova N, Trajkovski Z, et al. Congenital lipomatous overgrowth, vascular malformations, and epidermal nevi (CLOVE) syndrome: CNS malformations and seizures may be a component of this disorder. Am J Med Genet A. 2008;146A(20):2688–90. PMCID: 2819374.
4. Kurek KC, Luks VL, Ayturk UM, Alomari AI, Fishman SJ, Spencer SA, Mulliken JB, Bowen ME, Yamamoto GL, Kozakewich HP, Warman ML. Somatic mosaic activating mutations in PIK3CA cause CLOVES syndrome. Am J Hum Genet. 2012;90(6):1108–15.
5. Happle R. Cutaneous manifestation of lethal genes. Hum Genet. 1986;72(3):280.
6. Happle R. Lethal genes surviving by mosaicism: a possible explanation for sporadic birth defects involving the skin. J Am Acad Dermatol. 1987;16(4):899–906.
7. Happle R. Klippel-Trenaunay syndrome: is it a paradominant trait? Br J Dermatol. 1993;128(4):465–6.
8. Samuels Y, Wang Z, Bardelli A, Silliman N, Ptak J, Szabo S, Yan H, Gazdar A, Powell SM, Riggins GJ, Willson JK, Markowitz S, Kinzler KW, Vogelstein B, Velculescu VE. High frequency of mutations of the PIK3CA gene in human cancers. Science. 2004;304(5670):554.
9. Biesecker LG, Happle R, Mulliken JB, Weksberg R, Graham Jr JM, Viljoen DL, et al. Proteus syndrome: diagnostic criteria, differential diagnosis, and patient evaluation. Am J Med Genet. 1999;84(5):389–95.
10. Lindhurst MJ, Sapp JC, Teer JK, Johnston JJ, et al. A mosaic activating mutation in AKT1 associated with the Proteus syndrome. N Engl J Med. 2011;365(7):611–9.
11. Gloviczki P, Hollier LH, Telander RL, Kaufman B, Bianco AJ, Stickler GB. Surgical implications of Klippel-Trenaunay syndrome. Ann Surg. 1983;197(3):353–62. PMCID: 1352741.
12. Garzon MC, Huang JT, Enjolras O, Frieden IJ. Vascular malformations. Part II: associated syndromes. J Am Acad Dermatol. 2007;56(4):541–64.

13. Timur AA, Driscoll DJ, Wang Q. Biomedicine and diseases: the Klippel-Trenaunay syndrome, vascular anomalies and vascular morphogenesis. Cell Mol Life Sci. 2005;62(13):1434–47.
14. Vikkula M, Boon LM, Mulliken JB. Molecular genetics of vascular malformations. Matrix Biol. 2001;20(5–6):327–35.
15. Aelvoet GE, Jorens PG, Roelen LM. Genetic aspects of the Klippel-Trenaunay syndrome. Br J Dermatol. 1992;126(6):603–7.
16. Whelan AJ, Watson MS, Porter FD, Steiner RD. Klippel-Trenaunay-Weber syndrome associated with a 5:11 balanced translocation. Am J Med Genet. 1995;59(4):492–4.
17. Wang Q, Timur AA, Szafranski P, Sadgephour A, Jurecic V, Cowell J, et al. Identification and molecular characterization of de novo translocation t(8;14)(q22.3;q13) associated with a vascular and tissue overgrowth syndrome. Cytogenet Cell Genet. 2001;95(3–4):183–8. PMCID: 1579861.
18. Timur AA, Sadgephour A, Graf M, Schwartz S, Libby ED, Driscoll DJ, et al. Identification and molecular characterization of a de novo supernumerary ring chromosome 18 in a patient with Klippel-Trenaunay syndrome. Ann Hum Genet. 2004;68(Pt 4):353–61.
19. Picascia DD, Esterly NB. Cutis marmorata telangiectatica congenita: report of 22 cases. J Am Acad Dermatol. 1989;20(6):1098–104.
20. South DA, Jacobs AH. Cutis marmorata telangiectatica congenita (congenital generalized phlebectasia). J Pediatr. 1978;93(6):944–9.
21. Kienast AK, Hoeger PH. Cutis marmorata telangiectatica congenita: a prospective study of 27 cases and review of the literature with proposal of diagnostic criteria. Clin Exp Dermatol. 2009;34(3):319–23.
22. Wroblewski I, Joannard A, Francois P, Baudain P, Beani JC, Beaudoing A. Cutis marmorata telangiectatica congenita with body asymmetry. Pediatrie. 1988;43(2):117–20.
23. Rogers M, Poyzer KG. Cutis marmorata telangiectatica congenita. Arch Dermatol. 1982;118(11):895–9.
24. Lapunzina P, Gairi A, Delicado A, Mori MA, Torres ML, Goma A, et al. Macrocephaly-cutis marmorata telangiectatica congenita: report of six new patients and a review. Am J Med Genet A. 2004;130A(1):45–51.
25. Kennedy C, Oranje AP, Keizer K, van den Heuvel MM, Catsman-Berrevoets CE. Cutis marmorata telangiectatica congenita. Int J Dermatol. 1992;31(4):249–52.
26. Danarti R, Happle R, Konig A. Paradominant inheritance may explain familial occurrence of Cutis marmorata telangiectatica congenita. Dermatology. 2001;203(3):208–11.
27. Wright DR, Frieden IJ, Orlow SJ, Shin HT, Chamlin S, Schaffer JV, et al. The misnomer "macrocephaly-cutis marmorata telangiectatica congenita syndrome": report of 12 new cases and support for revising the name to macrocephaly-capillary malformations. Arch Dermatol. 2009;145(3):287–93.
28. Robertson SP, Gattas M, Rogers M, Ades LC. Macrocephaly – cutis marmorata telangiectatica congenita: report of five patients and a review of the literature. Clin Dysmorphol. 2000;9(1):1–9.
29. Rivière JB, Mirzaa GM, O'Roak BJ, Beddaoui M, et al. De novo germline and postzygotic mutations in AKT3, PIK3R2 and PIK3CA cause a spectrum of related megalencephaly syndromes. Nat Genet. 2012;44(8):934–40.
30. Wu NF, Kushnick T. The Beckwith-Wiedemann syndrome. The exomphalos-macroglossia-gigantism syndrome. Clin Pediatr (Phila). 1974;13(5):452–7.
31. Weksberg R, Shuman C, Smith AC. Beckwith-Wiedemann syndrome. Am J Med Genet C: Semin Med Genet. 2005;137C(1):12–23.
32. Weksberg R, Smith AC, Squire J, Sadowski P. Beckwith-Wiedemann syndrome demonstrates a role for epigenetic control of normal development. Hum Mol Genet. 2003;12(Spec No 1):R61–8.
33. Choufani S, Shuman C, Weksberg R. Beckwith-Wiedemann syndrome. Am J Med Genet C: Semin Med Genet. 2010;154C(3):343–54.

34. Huang H, Potter CJ, Tao W, Li DM, Brogiolo W, Hafen E, et al. PTEN affects cell size, cell proliferation and apoptosis during Drosophila eye development. Development. 1999;126(23):5365–72.
35. Eng C, Marsh D, Liaw D, Dahia P, et al., editors. Germline mutations of the PTEN gene in Cowden disease and Bannayan-Zonana syndrome. 47th Annual American Society of Human Genetics meeting; 1997; Baltimore.
36. Gao X, Pan D. TSC1 and TSC2 tumor suppressors antagonize insulin signaling in cell growth. Genes Dev. 2001;15(11):1383–92. PMCID: 312704.
37. Marsh DJ, Dahia PL, Zheng Z, Liaw D, Parsons R, Gorlin RJ, et al. Germline mutations in PTEN are present in Bannayan-Zonana syndrome. Nat Genet. 1997;16(4):333–4.
38. Eng C. Will the real Cowden syndrome please stand up: revised diagnostic criteria. J Med Genet. 2000;37(11):828–30. PMCID: 1734465.
39. Lynch ED, Ostermeyer EA, Lee MK, Arena JF, Ji H, Dann J, et al. Inherited mutations in PTEN that are associated with breast cancer, Cowden disease, and juvenile polyposis. Am J Hum Genet. 1997;61(6):1254–60. PMCID: 1716102.
40. Liaw D, Marsh DJ, Li J, Dahia PL, Wang SI, Zheng Z, et al. Germline mutations of the PTEN gene in Cowden disease, an inherited breast and thyroid cancer syndrome. Nat Genet. 1997;16(1):64–7.
41. Arch EM, Goodman BK, Van Wesep RA, Liaw D, Clarke K, Parsons R, et al. Deletion of PTEN in a patient with Bannayan-Riley-Ruvalcaba syndrome suggests allelism with Cowden disease. Am J Med Genet. 1997;71(4):489–93.
42. Nelen MR, van Staveren WC, Peeters EA, Hassel MB, Gorlin RJ, Hamm H, et al. Germline mutations in the PTEN/MMAC1 gene in patients with Cowden disease. Hum Mol Genet. 1997;6(8):1383–7.
43. Lok C, Viseux V, Avril MF, Richard MA, Gondry-Jouet C, Deramond H, et al. Brain magnetic resonance imaging in patients with Cowden syndrome. Medicine (Baltimore). 2005;84(2):129–36.
44. Turnbull MM, Humeniuk V, Stein B, Suthers GK. Arteriovenous malformations in Cowden syndrome. J Med Genet. 2005;42(8), e50. PMCID: 1736111.
45. Tan WH, Baris HN, Burrows PE, Robson CD, Alomari AI, Mulliken JB, et al. The spectrum of vascular anomalies in patients with PTEN mutations: implications for diagnosis and management. J Med Genet. 2007;44(9):594–602. PMCID: 2597949.
46. Caux F, Plauchu H, Chibon F, Faivre L, Fain O, Vabres P, et al. Segmental overgrowth, lipomatosis, arteriovenous malformation and epidermal nevus (SOLAMEN) syndrome is related to mosaic PTEN nullizygosity. Eur J Hum Genet. 2007;15(7):767–73.
47. Lachlan KL, Lucassen AM, Bunyan D, Temple IK. Cowden syndrome and Bannayan Riley Ruvalcaba syndrome represent one condition with variable expression and age-related penetrance: results of a clinical study of PTEN mutation carriers. J Med Genet. 2007;44(9):579–85. PMCID: 2597943.
48. Boon LM, Mulliken JB, Vikkula M. RASA1: variable phenotype with capillary and arteriovenous malformations. Curr Opin Genet Dev. 2005;15(3):265–9.
49. Eerola I, Boon LM, Mulliken JB, Burrows PE, Dompmartin A, Watanabe S, et al. Capillary malformation-arteriovenous malformation, a new clinical and genetic disorder caused by RASA1 mutations. Am J Hum Genet. 2003;73(6):1240–9.
50. Revencu N, Boon LM, Mulliken JB, Enjolras O, Cordisco MR, Burrows PE, et al. Parkes Weber syndrome, vein of Galen aneurysmal malformation, and other fast-flow vascular anomalies are caused by RASA1 mutations. Hum Mutat. 2008;29(7):959–65.
51. Coelho CM, Leevers SJ. Do growth and cell division rates determine cell size in multicellular organisms? J Cell Sci. 2000;113(Pt 17):2927–34.
52. Montagne J, Stewart MJ, Stocker H, Hafen E, Kozma SC, Thomas G. Drosophila S6 kinase: a regulator of cell size. Science. 1999;285(5436):2126–9.
53. Maehama T, Dixon JE. The tumor suppressor, PTEN/MMAC1, dephosphorylates the lipid second messenger, phosphatidylinositol 3,4,5-trisphosphate. J Biol Chem. 1998;273(22): 13375–8.

54. Wu X, Senechal K, Neshat MS, Whang YE, Sawyers CL. The PTEN/MMAC1 tumor suppressor phosphatase functions as a negative regulator of the phosphoinositide 3-kinase/Akt pathway. Proc Natl Acad Sci U S A. 1998;95(26):15587–91. PMCID: 28087.
55. Potter CJ, Huang H, Xu T. Drosophila Tsc1 functions with Tsc2 to antagonize insulin signaling in regulating cell growth, cell proliferation, and organ size. Cell. 2001;105(3):357–68.
56. Barker KT, Houlston RS. Overgrowth syndromes: is dysfunctional PI3-kinase signalling a unifying mechanism? Eur J Hum Genet. 2003;11(9):665–70.

Chapter 3
Vasculogenesis and Angiogenesis

Chang Zoon Chun, Rashmi Sood, and Ramani Ramchandran

Introduction

The development of the circulatory system is one of the earliest events in organogenesis [1]. This system is comprised of interconnected tubes that form an intricate network for transporting blood and lymph across tissues. The endothelial cells (ECs) line the inner walls of the tubes, and vascular smooth muscle cells surround them on the outside. The circulatory system is comprised of two primary vessel types, namely, the blood vessels and the lymphatic vessels [2]. These vessels differ in the content of their lumen. Blood vessels primarily carry blood, while lymphatic vessels carry lymph fluid. Blood vessels are comprised of arteries and veins. Arteries carry oxygenated blood that flows under high pressure, while the veins carry deoxygenated blood back to the heart under low pressure. The dorsal aorta (DA) and cardinal vein (CV) are the first to arise in a developing embryo. These are formed de novo via the assembly of endothelial precursors into a primitive vascular network (or plexus) through a process called "vasculogenesis" [3]. Once the primitive vascular plexus is established, a complex remodeling process consisting of migration, proliferation, sprouting, and pruning ensues and leads to the development of a functional circulatory system. This remodeling process is referred to as

C.Z. Chun, PhD
Department of Medicine, Division of Nephrology, Hypertension, & Renal Transplantation, University of Florida, Gainesville, FL, USA

R. Sood, PhD (✉)
Department of Pathology, Medical College of Wisconsin, Inc., Milwaukee, WI, USA
e-mail: rsood@mcw.edu

R. Ramchandran, PhD (✉)
Departments of Pediatrics, and Obstetrics and Gynecology, Neonatology, Medical College of Wisconsin, Inc., Milwaukee, WI, USA
e-mail: rramchan@mcw.edu

© Springer Science+Business Media New York 2016
P.E. North, T. Sander (eds.), *Vascular Tumors and Developmental Malformations*, Molecular and Translational Medicine, DOI 10.1007/978-1-4939-3240-5_3

"angiogenesis" [4]. Small capillaries and the intersomitic vessels (ISVs; vessels that traverse early body segments or somites) are formed through the angiogenesis mechanism.

Embryonic programs of angiogenesis and vasculogenesis are recapitulated in the adult during repair and healing processes and in mammalian reproduction. Ovulation, menstruation, implantation, and placentation are critically dependent on angiogenesis and neovascularization. The placenta undergoes extensive vascular growth and remodeling throughout pregnancy. Vascularization of the placenta is unique in its requirement for coordinated development of maternal and fetal vessels. This allows formation of large surface areas of exchange between maternal and fetal circulations, necessary for placental function. Specialized placental cells, termed trophoblast cells, are involved in the regulation of this process. Inadequate or abnormal vascularization of the placenta impacts the start of life and has far-reaching consequences on the metabolic and cardiovascular health in adult life [5, 6]. Abnormal angiogenesis and neovascularization are also associated with other pathological conditions such as tumor growth. Tumors secrete EC stimulatory growth factors that induce the host vasculature to sprout and grow in an angiogenic fashion. The new vessels are used by the tumor to traverse to distant sites, thus promoting metastases. In this chapter, we will discuss the basic principles governing vasculogenesis and angiogenesis in the embryo and placenta. In addition, we will discuss the molecules involved in these processes and the role that they play in the development of vascular anomalies.

Origin of Cells of the Vascular Lineage

All tissues of the body emerge from the three germ layers of ectoderm, endoderm, and mesoderm. Post gastrulation, the mesoderm germ layer gives rise to cells of the heart, kidney, muscle, and blood-forming tissues in addition to the cells of the circulatory system, namely, the vascular ECs. The vascular ECs emerge from the lateral most region of the mesoderm termed as the lateral plate mesoderm (LPM). The specification step from the LPM to the precursor cells of the vascular lineage is poorly understood. One putative intermediate step in this specification pathway is the formation of a bipotential precursor cell from the LPM that has capabilities to differentiate into the vascular and hematopoietic lineage. Evidence for the existence of such a bipotential precursor cell is observed during embryonic development, especially in the extraembryonic mouse yolk sac "blood islands"; these are loose aggregates of blood cells surrounded by the endothelium [7]. The outer cells of the blood island clusters appear flattened and subsequently differentiate into ECs, whereas the inner cells become hematopoietic cells [8]. In mouse embryo, this precursor cell is mainly located in the primitive streak (thickening region of the embryo showing noticeable first stages of development) and is only detectable for a very brief period of time [9] and eventually expresses *CD31*, *flk-1*, *flt-1*, and *tie-2* [10] markers, which are characteristic of EC lineage. Similarly, in chick, *flk-1*+ cells (Quek1) are abundant in the mesoderm that exits from the posterior primitive streak during gastrulation [11]. These cells contribute to the formation of both embryonic and extraembryonic mesoderm tissue, which gives rise to the first blood islands [12]. Gene targeting experiments in mouse demonstrate that a functional Flk-1 receptor tyrosine kinase is required for the development of the blood islands, providing further evidence that both hematopoietic and endothelial lineages are derived from a common precursor [13]. This common precursor cell is referred to as hemangioblast, which will be discussed in detail in the next section.

The Case for Hemangioblast

Nearly a century ago, based on observations in chick embryos that both hematopoietic and ECs are closely situated and develop together, a new term called "hemangioblast" was proposed to describe the common precursor cell [14, 15] that gives rise to both lineages. In terms of model systems, zebrafish has contributed immensely to our understanding of hemangioblast because of the identification of the first genetic mutant in vertebrate, "*cloche*," which lacks both ECs and blood cells suggesting that the mutation lies in the critical gene (as yet unidentified) that specifies the critical dual potential hemangioblast cell to vascular and blood lineage [16, 17]. More recently, Vogeli and his group constructed single-cell-resolution fate maps that show individual cells in zebrafish late blastula and gastrula can give rise to both hematopoietic and ECs [18]. Substantial characterization of the hemangioblasts has occurred in vitro through the utilization of the embryonic stem cell (ESC)-derived embryoid body (EB) model system. In the mouse and human ESC-derived EB cultures, single blast colony-forming cells (BL-CFCs) generate colonies that contain both hematopoietic and ECs. These cells emerge in the presence of VEGF-A and bone morphogenetic protein-4 (BMP-4) [10, 19, 20]. Further, they express *flk-1* and the mesodermal marker *brachyury* [21]. Based on the ability of genetically engineered ESCs to differentiate into BL-CFCs in vitro, *flk-1*, *Scl*, *Runx-1*, *Hhex*, *Mixl-1*, *Bmp-4*, *Smad-1*, *Gata-2*, and *Lycat* have all been shown to be essential for the generation of BL-CFCs [22–31]. In addition to these genes, *Lmo*, *fli-1*, and *etsrp* have been recently implicated in the specification of hemangioblast from the posterior LPM in zebrafish [32–37]. Importantly, constitutive activation of *fli1* is shown to be sufficient to induce expression of key hemangioblast genes such as *scl*, *lmo*, *gata2*, *etsrp*, and *flk-1* [38]. At present, our knowledge of hemangioblast specification from LPM is emerging; however, our knowledge downstream of hemangioblast is better known, as will be discussed in the next section.

Vasculogenesis Mechanisms in the Developing Embryo

The hemangioblast cell can differentiate down either the vascular lineage or the hematopoietic lineage. If the program for vascular lineage differentiation is initiated, the hemangioblast becomes more differentiated, and this cell type is called angioblast. The great vessels of the developing embryo such as the aorta and vein are formed directly from this cell population via a process of vasculogenesis [39]. The essential steps in vasculogenesis post angioblast specification are the migration of angioblasts toward the location of future developing vessels, the coalescence of precursor cells to tube formation, and the final maturation of vessels to establish functional circulation [40–42].

Both mice and zebrafish have extensively contributed to our knowledge of vasculogenesis. In mice, the first intraembryonic angioblasts are seen as early as 1 somite (som) stage at the lateral edges of the anterior intestinal portal and ventral to the somites [43]. In zebrafish, angioblasts are observed as early as 1 som in the LPM. An ets-related transcription factor protein (*etsrp or etv2*) was recently shown to be necessary and sufficient for angioblast specification at the LPM [36] and serves as a marker of angioblasts in the developing embryo. Moreover, *etsrp* is induced by *fli1* transcription factor [38], therefore implying that *fli1* is upstream of *etsrp*. Therefore, double positive *fli+/etsrp+* cells are used as pre-migratory vascular precursor cells (FEVPs) that are ideal for cell tracking during the vasculogenesis processes in zebrafish embryos. The *etsrp* cells in the head, trunk, and tail of a developing zebrafish follow unique patterns of movement, trajectory, and congregation that highlight the complex series of events that occurs when angioblasts are moving from the LPM to the midline. This unprecedented observation illuminates a highly organized series of events that are dictated by spatial and temporal cues [44].

The vasculogenesis process in zebrafish occurs in multiple stages: initially at pre-10 som stage followed by post-10 som stage. A cartoon is depicted in Fig. 3.1 that describes these events. During pre-10 som stage, the FEVPs increase in number at the LPM (at 10 som), and this increase is attributed to a proliferative mechanism that involves the Shh-vascular endothelial growth factor (VEGF)-Notch-Hey2 signaling pathway [44]. It is noteworthy that the number of angioblasts is not critical for their next step in vasculogenesis [45], i.e., migration to midline. At post-10 som stage (10–12 som), angioblast migration starts from the LPM toward the midline, which is in part controlled by signals from the endoderm [45]. At the midline, angioblasts first aggregate to form cord-like structures with no cell-cell junctions established, thereby resembling a poorly organized cluster of cells. However, for angioblast coalescence at the midline to occur effectively, cell-cell junctions need to form first, which occurs at ~17 hpf (16 som) in zebrafish [45]. In addition to cell-cell junctions, adherens junctions are also formed at this stage indicating that angioblasts are in close contact with each other. The next step in vasculogenesis is the coalescence of angioblasts to lumen formation in axial vessels (DA and PCV), which is poorly understood. An EC-derived secreted factor Egfl-7 was identified to regulate vascular tube formation in zebrafish [46], but the mechanisms involved in this process are not clear. A recent study proposes intracellular vacuolization as a proposed model for endothelial tube formation in vivo [47], but this mechanism was shown for smaller vessels and is not clear if it is applicable to larger vessels such as the primary axial vessels (DA and PCV) [45].

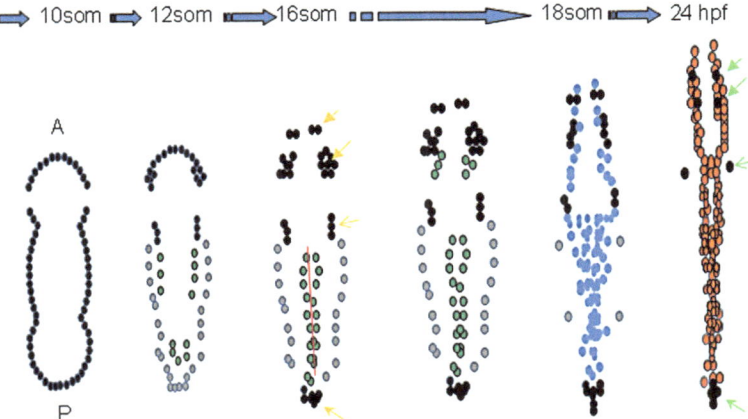

Fig. 3.1 *Etsrp⁺* angioblast cell development in zebrafish embryo. *Etsrp⁺* angioblasts appear in head, trunk lateral plate mesoderm (LPM), and tail region at 3 to 10 somite (som) embryos. The head region and the trunk LPM angioblasts contribute to cranial vessels and trunk axial vessels, respectively, during early embryonic vasculogenesis. At 12 to 16 som, head angioblasts show an inward trajectory resulting in four cephalic patches. At the same developmental stages, trunk LPM angioblasts show two distinct populations, anterior and posterior angioblasts. The anterior cells do not undergo substantial change. In contrast, posterior cells (*green circle*, 12 to 16 som) show coordinated movements such as the migration to the midline in an anterior to posterior direction in the trunk. At this time point, four distinct clusters of cells indicated by *yellow arrows* are evident along the axis of the embryo. At 18 som, most of angioblasts (*blue circle*) are closer to the midline in the trunk. At 18 to 20 som, the anterior trunk and the midline angioblasts come together at the site of future lateral dorsal aorta (DA). At 24 hpf, two major axial vessels, dorsal aorta (DA) and posterior cardinal vein (PCV), are observed (*brown circles*), and residual *etsrp⁺* cell (*green arrows*) remains for the next few hours

Artery vs. Vein (A/V) Specification Mechanisms in Developing Embryo

Once the primary vessels are formed, they take an identity of an artery or vein. Until recently, it was thought that flow dictated artery vs. vein (A/V) formation of primitive vessels [48, 49]. However, recent evidence shows that molecularly, artery and veins are fundamentally distinct in the early embryo thereby challenging the existing paradigm [50]. The embryonic expression pattern of ligand ephrin-B2 (efnb2) (specifically in artery ECs but not in venous ECs) prior to the onset of circulation in mouse embryos and its cognate receptor Ephrin-b4 (Ephb4) (expressed more in vein and less in artery) opened the door for identifying molecular markers that define arterial and venous cell identity [50]. At present, several artery- and vein-specific genes have been identified in vertebrate embryos [51, 52].

During the vasculogenesis process, the specification of angioblasts into artery or venous ECs is a critical step in the formation of arteries and veins, respectively [50]. In zebrafish, the differentiation of angioblasts into arterial and venous ECs first occurs at 17 hpf (16 som) [45]. The sonic hedgehog (Shh)-VEGF-Notch pathway is involved in A/V specification [52, 53], and a model is proposed to explain how and when A/V specification occurs in vivo. In this model, *shh* expressed in midline notochord cells induces medioventral somites to express VEGF. Because of this VEGF gradient, angioblasts migrate medially toward the midline [53]. VEGF over-expression in *shh*-deficient embryos induces arterial marker *efnb2* but not in *Notch-induced* embryos thereby placing VEGF downstream of Shh but upstream of Notch in arterial differentiation pathway [53]. Similarly in mice, VEGF and its isoforms promote arterial differentiation by inducing *efnb2*-positive vessels [54, 55]. Notch, downstream of VEGF, induces arterial-specific genes such as *efnb2* and represses venous-specific genes such as *flt-4* resulting in A/V specification [56]. Zebrafish embryos with reduced Notch activity have poorly formed DA and PCV often leading to arteriovenous malformation [56]. The hairy-and-enhancer-of-split-related (hey) family of transcription factors is a direct target of the Notch pathway [57]. In zebrafish, the *hey-2* genetic mutant *gridlock (grl)* [58] shows abnormal fusion of the lateral DA leading to aortic coarctation, a cardiovascular defect observed in humans [59]. Although *grl* expression is restricted to DA in zebrafish embryos, it does not appear to play a role in repressing venous markers such as *flt-4*, which might be mediated by another member of the hey family. Interestingly, in the grl^{m145} allele, arterial differentiation is normal, and defects in trunk vessel patterning are apparent suggesting that grl functions in the formation of DA, but its role in differentiation of artery ECs is unclear [52, 58, 60, 61]. Besides hey transcription factors (TF), members of FoxC TF family FoxC1 and FoxC2 are also involved in A/V specification. FoxC1/C2 upregulates the expression of *notch-1*, *notch-4*, and arterial markers *efnb2* and notch target *hey-2* [62] in mouse embryonic ECs suggesting that FoxC TF functions upstream of Notch to promote arterial specification.

In terms of signaling mechanisms, the mitogen-activated protein kinase (MAPK) and phosphoinositide-3-kinase (PI3K) pathways downstream of Flk-1 have been implicated as integral biochemical pathways for A/V specification [63]. Blocking of PI3K signaling pathway and activation of extracellular signal-regulated kinase-1 and kinase-2 (ERK-1/2) MAPK promote arterial fate, and conversely, activation of PI3K and blocking of ERK activation promote venous fate [63]. Compared to arterial specification, less emphasis has been placed on venous specification markers. Of the venous markers, the chicken ovalbumin upstream promoter-transcription factor II (COUP-TFII) is the best studied and is a member of the orphan nuclear receptor family that has been shown to actively maintain the venous state by inhibiting Notch activation [64].

Lymphatic Vessel Specification

Like A/V formation, the origins of lymphatics were controversial, until recent evidence conclusively shows that lymphatic ECs are specified from venous ECs [65, 66]. Similar to arteries and veins emerging from dual potential angioblasts, lymphatic cells emerge from dual potential venous ECs. Prox-1, a transcription factor, initiates lymphatic specification by expressing in a subset of bipotential venous ECs that differentiate into LECs [67, 68]. Prox-1 is also required for maintenance of lymphatic cell identity [69]. Recent work suggests that Sox-18 transcription factor may in part be responsible for inducing *prox-1* expression [70], thereby placing Sox-18 upstream of Prox-1. The Sox-18-induced *prox-1* expression commits dual potential venous cells to the lymphatic lineage. In addition to Prox-1 and Sox-18, Notch, FoxC2, and Efnb2 molecules that are involved in arterial specification are also involved in lymphatic specification [71]. In humans and mice, *Notch1* and *Notch4* are expressed in the lymphatics [72], and Notch signaling directly regulates VEGFR-3 expression in blood ECs [72]. Of the five isoforms of VEGF, VEGF-C is widely considered to mediate lymphatic sprouting through signals triggered on binding to cognate tyrosine kinase receptor VEGFR-3 in lymphatic ECs. FoxC2, transcription factor (TF) of the forkhead family, is also critical for lymphatic development, is expressed by LECs, and functions in lymphatic differentiation [73]. Loss of FoxC2 in mice results in failure to form lymphatic valves, abnormal accumulation of SMC to the lymphatic vasculature, and lymphatic dysfunction [74]. In terms of ephrins, mice at postnatal day 0 (P0) express both *efnb2* and *Ephb4* in dermal lymphatic vasculature [75]. Efnb2 signals via the intracellular PDZ domain, and deletion of the Efnb2 PDZ domain in mice results in lymphatic defects. These include defective dermal lymphatic remodeling, absence of lymphatic valves, abnormal accumulation of SMC in lymphatic capillaries, and chylothorax [75]. These defects suggest a role for efnb2 signaling in lymphangiogenesis.

Angiogenesis Along the Embryonic Body Axis

In the developing embryo, once the great vessels of the embryo, namely, DA and CV, are formed, secondary vasculature is initiated via an angiogenic mechanism. Zebrafish, chickens, and mice have extensively contributed to our understanding of this process. However, recently, zebrafish studies have provided mechanistic-based evidence of the angiogenesis process in vivo especially in the trunk region [76–78]. In the embryonic zebrafish trunk, vessels that traverse the somite (early muscle) boundaries are formed via the angiogenic process and are referred to as intersomitic vessels (ISVs). The ISVs in zebrafish form by discrete steps, and they first sprout from the established DA in pairs and align along the dorsoventral axis. The dorsalmost cell in the sprouting ISVs is called the "tip cell" or "leading cell," which progressively navigates through intersomitic boundaries and traverses the length of the chevron-like somites to join with its anterior and posterior neighbors, thus establishing a dorsal longitudinal anastomotic vessel (DLAVs). Interestingly, recent evidence shows the involvement of macrophage cells in linking the adjoining DLAVs in zebrafish and mice [79, 80]. Previously, it was thought that ISVs are comprised of three cells [81], but recent evidence shows that ISVs are comprised of multiple cells that overlap extensively to form a multicellular tube [77]. Recent data from

Blum et al. [77] suggest that ISVs lumen formation is a multicellular process containing an extracellular lumen with adjoining ISVs connected with tight junctions. Also, ISVs show a number of cellular behaviors including cell divisions, cell rearrangements, and dynamic changes in cell-cell contacts [77] that were previously unknown.

The mechanisms utilized for ISV formation are similar to another branching network, the nerves. In vertebrate ontogeny, the neural and vascular networks develop side-by-side [82] and utilize the branching processes of axons and blood vessels, respectively, to penetrate different regions of the body. Axons travel great distances to innervate tissues, while vessels travel shorter distances to perfuse tissues. A growing axon projects a sensory structure called a "growth cone" that integrates directional information provided by attraction and repulsion cues from the surrounding environment. Recent evidence suggests that capillaries sprout similarly from specialized ECs called "tip cells" [83]. Similar to the growth cone, the tip cell is a highly motile structure that constantly extends and retracts filopodia. The original idea came from retinal tip cells [83], which were thought not to proliferate but only provide guidance to the following stalk cell. However, ISVs' tip cells in zebrafish [77] do proliferate suggesting that tip cells from different tissue beds may have different functions. The VEGF and Notch family members participate in the tip vs. stalk cell positioning during angiogenic sprouting [84, 85]. Recent evidence suggests that relative levels of VEGF2 and VEGFR1, cognate receptors for VEGF, dictate which cell becomes a tip cell [86]. Guidance decisions of axons and tip cells are relayed by shared mechanisms at a molecular level [82], and members of the axon guidance molecule family, namely, *ephrins*, *semaphorins*, *netrins*, and *slits* along with their cognate receptors, work cooperatively to guide axonal growth cone pathfinding and vascular development (10) and are reviewed elsewhere [82].

Angiogenesis and Vasculogenesis in Placental Development

In mammals, angiogenic processes are recapitulated in the adult female during reproductive cycle and in pregnancy. The requirement for rapid and extensive neovascularization and remodeling perhaps makes the placenta the most active site of physiological angiogenesis and vasculogenesis. In this section, we discuss the unique aspects of blood vessel formation in the context of hemochorial placentation. This type of placentation is observed in humans, apes, and rodents and is characterized by direct contact of maternal blood with cells of fetal origin. While in all other organs blood flows through tubes of ECs, in the hemochorial placenta, maternal blood flows through channels formed by specialized fetal cells, the trophoblast cells (Fig. 3.2f). Trophoblast cells arise from the extraembryonic epithelium and are a unique cell type of the placenta. They play a critical role in regulating uterine vascular remodeling and fetoplacental vascularization. The next few paragraphs outline the processes involved in the establishment of maternal and fetal circulation in the hemochorial placenta and the regulatory role of trophoblast cells. For ease of

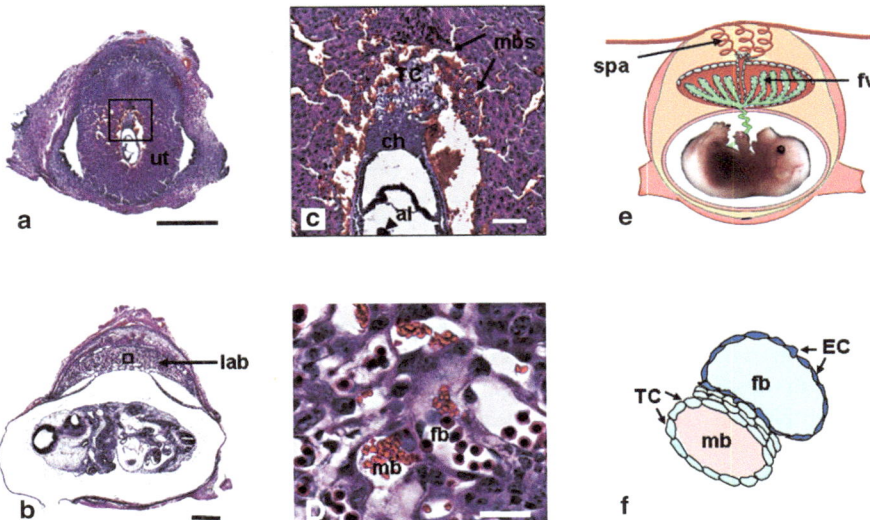

Fig. 3.2 Histological sections and schematic of murine placenta illustrating sites of angiogenesis and vasculogenesis in hemochorial placentation. Hematoxylin-eosin-stained sections of day 7.5 (**a**, **c**) and day 12.5 (**b**, **d**) placenta and schematic drawings of 12.5 placenta (**e**) and an area of placental labyrinth (**f**) are shown. (**c**) and (**d**) are enlarged images of boxed regions in (**a**) and (**b**). Angiogenesis and vascular remodeling in the uterine wall (ut) results in opening of maternal blood sinuses (mbs) to trophoblast cells (TC) surrounding the implanted embryo. The allantois (al) extended by the embryo meets the chorionic plate (ch) of trophoblast stem cells, initiating tropho-blast differentiation. Trophoblast lineages exposed to maternal blood adopt EC-like gene expression profile. Spiral arteries (spa) lose their endothelial and smooth muscle layers and convert to low resistance vessels, a process completed by invasion of trophoblast cells into the spiral arteries. Fetal vessels form de novo in the placenta through vasculogenesis in mesodermal cells of fetal villi (fv). Branching morphogenesis and angiogenesis result in the elaboration of fetal vasculature and formation of placental labyrinth (lab). The labyrinth is the site of exchange between fetal blood (fb) and maternal blood (mb). Trophoblast cells (TC) line maternal blood spaces. In contrast, fetal blood vessels are formed from endothelial cells (ECs). The process of fetoplacental vascularization is intimately linked to trophoblast differentiation. Scale bars represent 1 mm (**a**, **b**), 100 μm (**c**), and 25 μm (**d**), respectively. Note that the schematics are not meant to be anatomically accurate

discussion, these processes have been grouped as (1) uterine angiogenesis and vascular remodeling, (2) trophoblast differentiation and pseudovasculogenesis, and (3) fetoplacental vascularization.

The uterus (the organ where the embryo implants) undergoes several changes postconception. These changes, broadly termed as decidualization, include *uterine angiogenesis* and *vascular remodeling*. Uterine angiogenesis is initiated before, and continues after, implantation or the attachment of the blastocyst to the uterus. Trophoblast cells present in the outermost layer of the conceptus mediate this attachment. In rodents, initial uterine angiogenesis involves degeneration of epithelial cells surrounding the implantation chamber; changes in morphology of arterial capillaries in the vicinity, such that their lumens are enlarged and walls become thin to resemble sinusoids, and hypertrophy of ECs lining these sinusoids [87–89]. As a result of these processes, an anastomosing network of maternal blood sinuses surrounds the implantation chamber and fetal trophoblast cells (Fig. 3.2a, c). In rodents, around 8 days post coitum (dpc), some of the sinusoids open into the implantation chamber and bathe fetal trophoblast cells with maternal blood.

As pregnancy proceeds beyond 9 dpc (corresponding to the end of the first trimester in human pregnancy), the placenta undergoes tremendous growth at a rapid rate. In preparation for this growth, in addition to vascular adaptations at the feto-maternal interface, changes are necessary in larger vessels supplying the uterus. These include significant increases in diameter and length and changes in extracellular matrix composition of arteries that supply the uterus [90]. Extensive remodeling is observed in spiral arteries within the uterus (Fig. 3.2e). The endothelium and smooth muscle layers of uterine spiral arteries are disrupted and replaced by invading trophoblast cells [91]. The net result of these changes is reduced resistance of uterine arteries and an increased and privileged blood supply to the placenta.

Various molecular events involved in uterine angiogenesis and decidualization have been identified [92]. These are regulated by steroid hormones, estrogen and progesterone, and by prostaglandins [93, 94]. Similar to embryonic angiogenesis, VEGF and its receptor VEGFR-2 have also been identified as important mediators of uterine angiogenesis [94, 95]. Angiogenesis can proceed to a large extent with mechanical stimulation of hormonally primed uteri (without blastocyst implantation), suggesting a maternal hormonal control independent of direct regulation by fetal cells. It is, however, clear that fetal trophoblast cells also contribute to uterine angiogenesis. This is exemplified by the observation that abnormal hormonal expression by trophoblast cells in *Gata-2* or *Gata-3* knockout blastocysts implanted in heterozygous mothers (with normal gene expression) results in reduced uterine neovascularization [96]. Similar to uterine angiogenesis, the remodeling of spiral arteries is initiated when trophoblast cells are absent from its vicinity, but requires trophoblast invasion to proceed normally. Among other factors, maternal uterine natural killer cells play an important role in spiral artery remodeling (review [97]).

Trophoblast differentiation and *pseudovasculogenesis* comprise a second group of events intimately coupled with placental vascularization. About 70 % of the mature rodent placenta is made up of zygote-derived trophoblast cells [98]. They regulate many aspects of maternal vascular adaptation to pregnancy and provide the main structural and functional components needed to bring maternal and fetal blood systems in close contact (reviews [99, 100]). The trophoblast cell lineage is specified even before the embryo implants on the uterine wall. In mice, it appears as a sphere of epithelial cells, the trophectoderm, surrounding the inner cell mass and the blastocoel. Trophoblast cells depend on their interactions with embryonic tissues for continued proliferation and regulated differentiation [101]. Cells in direct contact with the inner cell mass maintain the trophoblast stem cell phenotype and form the chorionic plate (extraembryonic ectoderm). These later differentiate and form the bulk of the chorioallantoic placenta in a process initiated by fusion of the allantois (extraembryonic mesoderm extended by the embryo proper) with the chorionic plate (Fig. 3.2c). In mice, chorioallantoic fusion occurs around 8.5 dpc. Almost immediately, trophoblast differentiation is seen as the expression of *gcm1* in clusters of trophoblast cells in the chorionic plate. The chorion folds into branches initiated at sites of *gcm1* expression [102]. As the fetoplacental vasculature elaborates from the extraembryonic mesoderm filling these branches, trophoblast cells differentiate to form three distinct cell layers surrounding fetal vessels. Gene expression pattern in the early chorion suggests that trophoblast subtypes of these layers may be specified soon after chorioallantoic fusion [103]. Gene knockout studies and tetraploid aggregation assays have led to the identification of a number of genes that regulate trophoblast differentiation [99, 100]. By disrupting specific genes in the trophoblast compartment, their effects on placental development have been evaluated. These studies have underscored a critical role of trophoblast cell differentiation in fetoplacental vascularization.

As alluded to above, distinct subtypes of trophoblast cells constitute the placenta. They have been classified based on their origin, location in the placenta, and gene expression [26, 103–106]. Of these, trophoblast giant cells (TGCs), named after the large size of their polyploid nucleus, are the first to terminally differentiate. Based on their anatomic location, TGCs are thought to play an important role in uterine vascular remodeling. In the murine placenta, for example, at least four subtypes of TGCs occupy the blood-tissue interface [26, 103, 104]. These include spiral artery-associated TGCs (equivalent to endovascular trophoblasts in humans) that invade uterine spiral arteries and replace maternal ECs. In human pregnancies, shallow invasion by trophoblast cells is associated with incomplete remodeling of spiral arteries and obstetric syndromes of preeclampsia and intrauterine growth retardation [107, 108]. It has been further noted that invading trophoblast cells downregulate the expression of adhesion receptors characteristic of epithelial cells and begin to express EC-specific repertoire of adhesion receptors [109, 110]. This process has been termed as endothelial mimicry or *pseudovasculogenesis* and has been found to be incomplete or defective in preeclamptic pregnancies. More recent studies have shown that anticoagulant gene expression, characteristic of ECs, is also widely observed in trophoblast cells [111–113] and that trophoblast differentiation may be programmatically coupled to the acquisition of an EC-like anticoagulant gene expression profile [113]. Thus, the ability to mimic endothelial gene expression is not limited to the subpopulation of trophoblast cells that invade spiral arteries, but rather extends to trophoblast cells resident in the placenta. Trophoblast pseudovasculogenesis is likely to play an important role in the development and maintenance of an effective maternal circulation in the hemochorial placenta.

Trophoblast differentiation is regulated by several growth factors including activin, EGF, TGFβ, IGF-I, IGF-II, and PTHrP [106]. Upon differentiation, trophoblast cells produce a number of angiogenic hormones and their receptors, as well as vasoactive factors and proteases capable of mediating cellular degradation. These include proteins in the prolactin and growth hormone family, the VEGF gene family, adrenomedullin, endothelial nitric oxide synthase, and members of the cathepsin family of proteases [106, 114–116]. The expression of these factors is spatially and temporally restricted and often associated with certain subtypes of trophoblast cells. Subsets of trophoblast cells also express alternately spliced form of VEGFR-1, a secreted protein also called sFlt-1, which blocks VEGF action. Expression of sFlt-1 by trophoblast cells is thought to be a part of mechanisms by which fetal cells regulate excessive uterine angiogenesis and prevent maternal vessels from growing into the placental junctional zone [117, 118].

Concomitant with trophoblast differentiation, development of fetal vessels in the placenta, termed as *fetoplacental vascularization*, is also initiated with the formation of the chorioallantoic placenta. The fusion of the allantois with the chorion initiates branching morphogenesis at sites of *gcm1* expression. The trophoblast branches get filled with allantoic mesoderm from which the stromal and vascular components of the fetal placenta arise [102, 103, 119]. Fetal vessels in the placenta are formed de novo from hemangiogenic precursors that arise from the mesenchyme of fetal villi (Fig. 3.2e) rather than sprouting of vessels from the embryo into the placenta. Morphologically distinct CD34$^+$ cells can be observed forming primitive cords in human placental villi as early as day 22 of pregnancy [120]. Continuous branching morphogenesis and angiogenic processes produce a complex structure with a large surface area of exchange with maternal blood sinuses (Fig. 3.2d–f).

The molecular regulators and pathways of fetoplacental vascularization are thought to be similar to those identified for vascularization of the embryo (review [121]). Angiogenesis factors expressed in the allantoic mesoderm include members of VEGF and fibroblast growth factor (FGF) gene families and their receptors [122–125]. Gene knockout studies in mice suggest that these may be involved in vascularization of the yolk sac and, by extension, the allantoic mesoderm [122, 124, 126–128]. Fetoplacental vascularization also involves mechanisms regulated by trophoblast cells. It is clear that trophoblast branching morphogenesis is essential for fetoplacental vascularization. Mice mutants affected in branching morphogenesis are simultaneously affected in fetoplacental vascularization, although the location of primary defect is not very clear [100]. Angiogenic and anti-angiogenic factors secreted by trophoblast cells are candidate mechanisms involved in regulation of fetoplacental vascularization [116, 129, 130].

Abnormal Placental Vascularization and Pregnancy Complications

Optimal vascularization and blood flow are critical for placental function. Defective or inadequate maternal spiral artery remodeling, thrombotic lesions in maternal and fetal vasculature, and benign placental vascular tumors, such as chorioangiomas, are the most common types of pathologies affecting placental blood flow. Depending on the severity of defect, these placental vasculopathies are associated with increased risk of pregnancy complications affecting maternal health and fetal development. While severe defects result in fetal loss, continuation of pregnancy with suboptimal placental function is associated with fetal growth restriction and maternal hypertensive disorders, such as preeclampsia. In rodents, suppression of angiogenesis reduces fetal and placental size and causes hypertension in the mother [131, 132]. Administration of anti-angiogenic factors such as the soluble form of VEGFR-1 (sVEGFR-1, also called sFlt-1) or the soluble form of TGF-β1 co-receptor, endoglin (sEng), in maternal circulation of pregnant rats leads to severe preeclampsia and fetal growth restriction [133, 134]. An accumulating body of evidence suggests that human pregnancies complicated with preeclampsia are also associated with changes in levels of angiogenic and anti-angiogenic factors in maternal circulation. These include increases in sFlt-1 and sEng levels and lowering of PIGF (placental growth factor), VEGF, and TGF-β1 [133, 135–137]. These findings have opened the possibility of using circulating levels of pro- and anti-angiogenic factors as early biomarkers of preeclampsia and restoring angiogenic balance with therapeutic agents [138]. Consistent with the highly angiogenic nature of the placenta and its ability to suppress inappropriate angiogenesis in adjacent maternal and fetal tissues, placenta has been implicated as the site of origin of infantile hemangiomas, discussed in the next section and in more detail in Chapter 1 [139].

Vascular Anomalies

Vascular anomalies are classified into two distinct groups: vascular tumors and vascular malformations. Infantile hemangioma, classified as a vascular tumor, is the most common tumor of infancy and develops within weeks after birth, rapidly proliferates during the first year of life via endothelial and pericytic hyperplasia, then slowly involutes over a period of years [140, 141]. Infantile hemangiomas share common immunomarkers and a genome-wide transcriptional similarity with placental ECs [139, 142]. This unique similarity, along with perinatal presentation, limited growth and eventual spontaneous involution has led to the hypothesis that infantile hemangiomas arise from embolized placental ECs that become dislodged into fetal circulation [139, 143]. A correlation has been observed between the incidence of infantile hemangiomas and premature birth, low birth weight, and maternal preeclampsia. Examination of a relationship between the presence of placental vascular abnormalities and the incidence of infantile hemangiomas is a matter of active research.

Vascular malformations on the other hand are present at birth, do not proliferate, but grow proportionately with the infant throughout the life of the individual [144]. They are thought to be inborn embryonic errors in vascular development. Vascular malformations are named according to the vessel type they affect. For example, venous malformations are those associated with veins, and lymphatic malformations are those associated with lymphatic vessels. The incidence of venous malformation is 1 in 10,000 [145]. Venous anomalies are subdivided into venous malformations (VM) and glomuvenous malformations (GVM). The majority of cases (95 %) fall into the VM category, which include sporadic VM and cutaneomucosal VM (VMCM), while GVM include 5 % of the cases [144]. The etiology of sporadic

VMs and syndromes such as Maffucci syndrome and Klippel-Trenaunay syndrome that are associated with VMs is unknown.

Besides histological classifications, vascular malformations can be classified according to hemodynamic features during angiography. For example, lymphatic and VMs are "low-flow" lesions, while arterial or arteriovenous malformations (AVMs) are "high-flow" lesions. AVMs have been postulated to result from the defective separation of uncommitted angioblasts as arteries and veins, i.e., impaired arterial specification/differentiation during blood vessel formation. Lymphatic malformations (LMs) may be focal or generalized. LMs usually enlarge slowly over time and often displace adjacent organs. The incidence rate of LMs is 1.2–2.8 per 1000 live births [146]. Despite their "benign" nature, vascular malformations present major medical challenges, both diagnostically and in terms of clinical management. Current therapies are limited in efficacy and have significant complications [147].

Genetic Causes of Vascular Malformations

Vascular malformations are usually focal and sporatic, without familial association. However, inheritance of vascular malformations in families has been observed. Sporadic forms often present with a single lesion, while multiple lesions are often observed in inherited forms. The prevailing hypothesis attributes familial forms of some types of vascular malformations to a "double-hit mechanism" where the primary hit is germline heterozygous resulting in incomplete penetrance, variable expressivity, and multifocality of lesions often observed in inherited VMs [144]. A second somatic hit either in the same gene or in a signaling pathway regulated by the primary hit results in full penetrance of the phenotype including multifocal lesions. Lymphatic malformations on the other hand are usually congenital with no evidence for inheritance, suggesting that somatic mutations in a restricted area of the lymphatic network result in lesions.

Significant advances have been made in identifying genetic and molecular determinants of a variety of vascular anomalies. Mutations in *TIE2* [145, 148] for multiple cutaneous and mucosal VMs, in *GLOMULIN* [149] for GVMs, and in *VEGFR-3*, *FOXC-2*, *NEMO*, and *SOX-18* for lymphedema or related syndromes have been identified [150]. For a more complete listing, see Chapter 4. The concept of somatic mutations as a possible cause for vascular anomalies although not absolute is definitely gaining strength. We recently identified mutations in two genes, namely, *sucrose non-fermenting-related kinase-1* (*SNRK-1*) and *dual-specific phosphatase-5* (*DUSP-5*) in patients with vascular anomalies [151]. *Snrk-1* and *Dusp-5* both participate together in controlling early endothelial precursor cell population in zebrafish. We have observed *DUSP-5* mutations, but not *SNRK-1* mutations, in infantile hemangioma. Because IH is characterized by initial rapid growth and eventual involution, we hypothesize that loss of *dusp-5* function may promote vascular precursor cell migration or growth during the tumor's proliferative phase. This may occur via the removal of *dusp-5*'s blockade of *snrk-1* signaling. Alternatively, *DUSP-5* mutations might promote endothelial apoptosis during involution because this has been observed in Dusp-5 loss-of-function differentiated ECs [151]. The coordination of *dusp-5* and *snrk-1* signaling in regulating angioblast numbers and migration in the zebrafish suggests that somatic mutations in either gene might cause or modulate congenital vascular malformations. We found *DUSP-5* mutations in 1 of 3 IH specimens and in 12 of 17 vascular and lymphatic malformations. All *DUSP-5* mutations observed in vascular anomaly specimens were not conservative substitutions, but ones that would alter protein structure, charge, and in turn, function. Thus, we conclude that alterations in Dusp-5 may be associated with a variety of vascular abnormalities.

Interestingly, the *SNRK-1* mutations observed were found exclusively in venous and lymphatic malformations, suggesting that loss of *SNRK-1* expression influences these vascular anomalies. The lymphatic vascular system develops from the venous system [152], and venous and lymphatic malformations are often mixed as was the case in 5 of 8 tissue specimens containing a *SNRK-1* mutation. Our data suggests that somatic mutations in *SNRK-1* and *DUSP-5* may be found in a minority of cells present in affected tissues, although direct evidence will be obtained from sequencing these genes from blood cells of these patients. Based on high expression of *SNRK-1* in infantile hemangioma tissue (Paula North & RR data not published), we hypothesize that the mutation is present in ECs or EC precursor population. However, its presence in other supporting cells such as mesenchyme [153] cannot be excluded. To better evaluate the clinical relevance of *SNRK-1* and *DUSP-5* mutations, future studies will focus on analyzing tissues from more patients with vascular anomalies and correlate our findings with clinical presentations. Nevertheless, our studies suggest that the pathogenesis of vascular malformations may be impacted by aberrant *dusp-5* and *snrk-1* signaling. Recently, reactive oxygen species have been reported to inhibit the catalytic activity of specific tyrosine phosphatases (Dusp-1) in an angiomyolipoma cell model [154] and treatment using nicotinamide adenine dinucleotide phosphate (reduced form) oxidase (Nox) inhibitors abolished tumor growth in vivo in a mouse model of hemangioma via blockage of angiopoietin-2 production [155]. Therefore, vascular anomaly therapy based on blocking aberrant kinases and phosphatases is an avenue worth exploring in the clinic.

Summary

The circulatory system is a critical component for a developing embryo. The cells of the circulatory system primarily originate from mesoderm tissue and more specifically from the LPM. Because blood cells and ECs emerge side-by-side from LPM, a common precursor cell, namely, hemangioblast that gives rise to both lineages, has been speculated. Hemangioblasts committed to a vascular lineage are called angioblasts. Angioblasts proliferate at LPM and migrate to midline where they coalesce to form the primary vessels of the embryo via a vasculogenic process.

During this process of migration to the midline, angioblasts differentiate into arteries and veins, and the Shh-Notch-VEGF-Notch signaling pathway is responsible for A/V specification. Once the primary vessels are formed, secondary vessels emerge, and those that emerge in the trunk region are called ISVs that are formed via an angiogenic process. The ISVs utilize axon guidance mechanisms and are guided by tip cells that sense local milieu, which directs the following stalk cell. Angiogenesis and vasculogenesis are rarely invoked in the adult, except during reproduction, wound healing, and in pathological conditions. The placenta is the site of most rapid and extensive neovascularization and remodeling observed in the adult. At the molecular level, angiogenic and vasculogenic mechanisms involved in placentation appear to recapitulate those observed during embryonic development. Vascularization of the placenta differs from other organs in its requirement for coordinated elaboration of maternal and fetal circulations that occurs in a matrix of trophoblast cells. Dysregulation of vascular growth control can result in formation of vascular anomalies. Several gene products have been identified to be mutated in vascular anomalies which, despite their "benign" nature, present major medical challenges, both diagnostically and in terms of clinical management. Current therapies are limited in efficacy and have significant complications. Identification of specific mutations in the lesions of individual patients will lead to better prediction of biological behaviors and outcomes and to the development of effective, targeted therapies.

References

1. Sabin FR. Studies on the origins of blood-vessels and of red blood corpuscles as seen in the living blastoderm of chicks during the second day of development. Contrib Embryol. 1920;36:213–62.
2. Sabin F. Studies on the origin of blood-vessels and of red blood corpuscles as seen in the living blastoderm of chicks on the second day of incubation. Contrib Embryol. 1920;36:213–61.
3. Risau W, Sariola H, Zerwes HG, Sasse J, Ekblom P, et al. Vasculogenesis and angiogenesis in embryonic-stem-cell-derived embryoid bodies. Development. 1988;102:471–8.
4. Hunter J (1787) Lectures on the principles of surgery. In: Palmer J, editor. The works of John Hunter, Haswell, Barrington and Haswell.
5. Barker DJ. In utero programming of chronic disease. Clin Sci (Lond). 1998;95:115–28.
6. Gluckman PD, Hanson MA. Living with the past: evolution, development, and patterns of disease. Science. 2004;305:1733–6.
7. Flamme I, Frolich T, Risau W. Molecular mechanisms of vasculogenesis and embryonic angiogenesis. J Cell Physiol. 1997;173:206–10.
8. Kessel J, Fabian BC. Graded morphogenetic patterns during the development of the extraembryonic blood system and coelom of the chick blastoderm: a scanning electron microscope and light microscope study. Am J Anat. 1985;173:99–112.
9. Huber TL, Kouskoff V, Fehling HJ, Palis J, Keller G. Haemangioblast commitment is initiated in the primitive streak of the mouse embryo. Nature. 2004;432:625–30.
10. Choi K, Kennedy M, Kazarov A, Papadimitriou JC, Keller G. A common precursor for hematopoietic and endothelial cells. Development. 1998;125:725–32.

11. Eichmann A, Marcelle C, Breant C, Le Douarin NM. Two molecules related to the VEGF receptor are expressed in early endothelial cells during avian embryonic development. Mech Dev. 1993;42:33–48.

12. Garcia-Martinez V, Schoenwolf GC. Primitive-streak origin of the cardiovascular system in avian embryos. Dev Biol. 1993;159:706–19.

13. Shalaby F, Ho J, Stanford WL, Fischer KD, Schuh AC, et al. A requirement for Flk1 in primitive and definitive hematopoiesis and vasculogenesis. Cell. 1997;89:981–90.

14. Sabin FR. Studies on the origin of blood vessels and of red corpuscles as seen in the living blastoderm of the chick during the second day of incubation: contributions to embryology. Contrib Embryol. 1920;9:213–62.

15. Murray PDF. The development in vitro of the blood of the early chick embryo. Proc R Soc Lond. 1932;111:497–521.

16. Stainier DY, Weinstein BM, Detrich 3rd HW, Zon LI, Fishman MC. Cloche, an early acting zebrafish gene, is required by both the endothelial and hematopoietic lineages. Development. 1995;121:3141–50.

17. Parker L, Stainier DY. Cell-autonomous and non-autonomous requirements for the zebrafish gene cloche in hematopoiesis. Development. 1999;126:2643–51.

18. Vogeli KM, Jin SW, Martin GR, Stainier DY. A common progenitor for haematopoietic and endothelial lineages in the zebrafish gastrula. Nature. 2006;443:337–9.

19. Kennedy M, D'Souza SL, Lynch-Kattman M, Schwantz S, Keller G. Development of the hemangioblast defines the onset of hematopoiesis in human ES cell differentiation cultures. Blood. 2007;109:2679–87.

20. Lu S-J, Feng Q, Caballero S, Chen Y, Moore MAS, et al. Generation of functional hemangioblasts from human embryonic stem cells. Nat Meth. 2007;4:501–9.

21. Fehling HJ, Lacaud G, Kubo A, Kennedy M, Robertson S, et al. Tracking mesoderm induction and its specification to the hemangioblast during embryonic stem cell differentiation. Development. 2003;130:4217–27.

22. Hidaka M, Stanford WL, Bernstein A. Conditional requirement for the Flk-1 receptor in the in vitro generation of early hematopoietic cells. Proc Natl Acad Sci U S A. 1999;96:7370–5.

23. Schuh AC, Faloon P, Hu QL, Bhimani M, Choi K. In vitro hematopoietic and endothelial potential of flk-1(–/–) embryonic stem cells and embryos. Proc Natl Acad Sci U S A. 1999;96:2159–64.

24. Faloon P, Arentson E, Kazarov A, Deng CX, Porcher C, et al. Basic fibroblast growth factor positively regulates hematopoietic development. Development. 2000;127:1931–41.

25. Robertson SM, Kennedy M, Shannon JM, Keller G. A transitional stage in the commitment of mesoderm to hematopoiesis requiring the transcription factor SCL/tal-1. Development. 2000;127:2447–59.

26. Chung YS, Zhang WJ, Arentson E, Kingsley PD, Palis J, et al. Lineage analysis of the hemangioblast as defined by FLK1 and SCL expression. Development. 2002;129:5511–20.

27. Lacaud G, Gore L, Kennedy M, Kouskoff V, Kingsley P, et al. Runx1 is essential for hematopoietic commitment at the hemangioblast stage of development in vitro. Blood. 2002;100:458–66.

28. Lacaud G, Kouskoff V, Trumble A, Schwantz S, Keller G. Haploinsufficiency of Runx1 results in the acceleration of mesodermal development and hemangioblast specification upon in vitro differentiation of ES cells. Blood. 2004;103:886–9.

29. Lugus JJ, Chung YS, Mills JC, Kim SI, Grass J, et al. GATA2 functions at multiple steps in hemangioblast development and differentiation. Development. 2007;134:393–405.

30. Wang C, Faloon PW, Tan Z, Lv Y, Zhang P, et al. Mouse lysocardiolipin acyltransferase controls the development of hematopoietic and endothelial lineages during in vitro embryonic stem-cell differentiation. Blood. 2007;110:3601–9.

31. Zafonte BT, Liu S, Lynch-Kattman M, Torregroza I, Benvenuto L, et al. Smad1 expands the hemangioblast population within a limited developmental window. Blood. 2007;109:516–23.

32. Gering M, Rodaway AR, Gottgens B, Patient RK, Green AR. The SCL gene specifies hae-mangioblast development from early mesoderm. EMBO J. 1998;17:4029–45.
33. Liao W, Ho CY, Yan YL, Postlethwait J, Stainier DY. Hhex and scl function in parallel to regulate early endothelial and blood differentiation in zebrafish. Development. 2000;127:4303–13.
34. Gering M, Yamada Y, Rabbitts TH, Patient RK. Lmo2 and Scl/Tal1 convert non-axial meso-derm into haemangioblasts which differentiate into endothelial cells in the absence of Gata1. Development. 2003;130:6187–99.
35. Dooley KA, Davidson AJ, Zon LI. Zebrafish scl functions independently in hematopoietic and endothelial development. Dev Biol. 2005;277:522–36.
36. Sumanas S, Lin S. Ets1-related protein is a key regulator of vasculogenesis in zebrafish. PLoS Biol. 2006;4, e10.
37. Patterson LJ, Gering M, Patient R. Scl is required for dorsal aorta as well as blood formation in zebrafish embryos. Blood. 2005;105:3502–11.
38. Liu F, Walmsley M, Rodaway A, Patient R. Fli1 acts at the top of the transcriptional network driving blood and endothelial development. Curr Biol. 2008;18:1234–40.
39. Poole TJ, Coffin JD. Vasculogenesis and angiogenesis: two distinct morphogenetic mecha-nisms establish embryonic vascular pattern. J Exp Zool. 1989;251:224–31.
40. Cleaver O, Krieg PA. VEGF mediates angioblast migration during development of the dorsal aorta in Xenopus. Development. 1998;125:3905–14.
41. Drake CJ, Fleming PA. Vasculogenesis in the day 6.5 to 9.5 mouse embryo. Blood. 2000;95:1671–9.
42. Ferguson 3rd JE, Kelley RW, Patterson C. Mechanisms of endothelial differentiation in embryonic vasculogenesis. Arterioscler Thromb Vasc Biol. 2005;25:2246–54.
43. Risau W, Flamme I. Vasculogenesis. Annu Rev Cell Dev Biol. 1995;11:73–91.
44. Chun CZ, Remadevi I, Schupp MO, Samant GV, Pramanik K, et al. Fli+ etsrp+ hemato-vascular progenitor cells proliferate at the lateral plate mesoderm during vasculogenesis in zebrafish. PLoS One. 2011;6:e14732.
45. Jin SW, Beis D, Mitchell T, Chen JN, Stainier DY. Cellular and molecular analyses of vascu-lar tube and lumen formation in zebrafish. Development. 2005;132:5199–209.
46. Parker LH, Schmidt M, Jin SW, Gray AM, Beis D, et al. The endothelial-cell-derived secreted factor Egfl7 regulates vascular tube formation. Nature. 2004;428:754–8.
47. Kamei M, Brian Saunders W, Bayless KJ, Dye L, Davis GE, et al. Endothelial tubes assemble from intracellular vacuoles in vivo. Nature. 2006;442:453–6.
48. Girard H. Arterial pressure in the chick embryo. Am J Physiol. 1973;224:454–60.
49. Gonzalez-Crussi F. Vasculogenesis in the chick embryo. An ultrastructural study. Am J Anat. 1971;130:441–60.
50. Wang HU, Chen ZF, Anderson DJ. Molecular distinction and angiogenic interaction between embryonic arteries and veins revealed by ephrin-B2 and its receptor Eph-B4. Cell. 1998;93:741–53.
51. Hirashima M, Suda T. Differentiation of arterial and venous endothelial cells and vascular morphogenesis. Endothelium. 2006;13:137–45.
52. Lawson ND, Weinstein BM. Arteries and veins: making a difference with zebrafish. Nat Rev Genet. 2002;3:674–82.
53. Lawson ND, Vogel AM, Weinstein BM. Sonic hedgehog and vascular endothelial growth factor act upstream of the Notch pathway during arterial endothelial differentiation. Dev Cell. 2002;3:127–36.
54. Visconti RP, Richardson CD, Sato TN. Orchestration of angiogenesis and arteriovenous con-tribution by angiopoietins and vascular endothelial growth factor (VEGF). Proc Natl Acad Sci U S A. 2002;99:8219–24.
55. Mukouyama YS, Shin D, Britsch S, Taniguchi M, Anderson DJ. Sensory nerves determine the pattern of arterial differentiation and blood vessel branching in the skin. Cell. 2002;109:693–705.

56. Lawson ND, Scheer N, Pham VN, Kim CH, Chitnis AB, et al. Notch signaling is required for arterial-venous differentiation during embryonic vascular development. Development. 2001;128:3675–83.

57. Iso T, Kedes L, Hamamori Y. HES and HERP families: multiple effectors of the Notch signaling pathway. J Cell Physiol. 2003;194:237–55.

58. Zhong TP, Rosenberg M, Mohideen MA, Weinstein B, Fishman MC. gridlock, an HLH gene required for assembly of the aorta in zebrafish. Science. 2000;287:1820–4.

59. Weinstein BM, Stemple DL, Driever W, Fishman MC. Gridlock, a localized heritable vascular patterning defect in the zebrafish. Nat Med. 1995;1:1143–7.

60. Zhong TP. Zebrafish genetics and formation of embryonic vasculature. Curr Top Dev Biol. 2005;71:53–81.

61. Zhong TP, Childs S, Leu JP, Fishman MC. Gridlock signalling pathway fashions the first embryonic artery. Nature. 2001;414:216–20.

62. Hayashi H, Kume T. Foxc transcription factors directly regulate Dll4 and Hey2 expression by interacting with the VEGF-Notch signaling pathways in endothelial cells. PLoS One. 2008;3, e2401.

63. Hong CC, Peterson QP, Hong JY, Peterson RT. Artery/vein specification is governed by opposing phosphatidylinositol-3 kinase and MAP kinase/ERK signaling. Curr Biol. 2006;16:1366–72.

64. You LR, Lin FJ, Lee CT, DeMayo FJ, Tsai MJ, et al. Suppression of Notch signalling by the COUP-TFII transcription factor regulates vein identity. Nature. 2005;435:98–104.

65. Yaniv K, Isogai S, Castranova D, Dye L, Hitomi J, et al. Imaging the developing lymphatic system using the zebrafish. Novartis Found Symp. 2007;283:139–48. discussion 148–151, 238–141.

66. Srinivasan RS, Dillard ME, Lagutin OV, Lin FJ, Tsai S, et al. Lineage tracing demonstrates the venous origin of the mammalian lymphatic vasculature. Genes Dev. 2007;21:2422–32.

67. Wigle JT, Oliver G. Prox1 function is required for the development of the murine lymphatic system. Cell. 1999;98:769–78.

68. Wigle JT, Harvey N, Detmar M, Lagutina I, Grosveld G, et al. An essential role for Prox1 in the induction of the lymphatic endothelial cell phenotype. EMBO J. 2002;21:1505–13.

69. Johnson NC, Dillard ME, Baluk P, McDonald DM, Harvey NL, et al. Lymphatic endothelial cell identity is reversible and its maintenance requires Prox1 activity. Genes Dev. 2008;22:3282–91.

70. Francois M, Caprini A, Hosking B, Orsenigo F, Wilhelm D, et al. Sox18 induces development of the lymphatic vasculature in mice. Nature. 2008;456:643–7.

71. Shawber CJ, Kitajewski J. Arterial regulators taken up by lymphatics. Lymphat Res Biol. 2008;6:139–43.

72. Shawber CJ, Funahashi Y, Francisco E, Vorontchikhina M, Kitamura Y, et al. Notch alters VEGF responsiveness in human and murine endothelial cells by direct regulation of VEGFR-3 expression. J Clin Invest. 2007;117:3369–82.

73. Seo S, Fujita H, Nakano A, Kang M, Duarte A, et al. The forkhead transcription factors, Foxc1 and Foxc2, are required for arterial specification and lymphatic sprouting during vascular development. Dev Biol. 2006;294:458–70.

74. Petrova TV, Karpanen T, Norrmen C, Mellor R, Tamakoshi T, et al. Defective valves and abnormal mural cell recruitment underlie lymphatic vascular failure in lymphedema distichiasis. Nat Med. 2004;10:974–81.

75. Makinen T, Adams RH, Bailey J, Lu Q, Ziemiecki A, et al. PDZ interaction site in ephrinB2 is required for the remodeling of lymphatic vasculature. Genes Dev. 2005;19:397–410.

76. Ellertsdottir E, Lenard A, Blum Y, Krudewig A, Herwig L, et al. Vascular morphogenesis in the zebrafish embryo. Dev Biol. 2010;341:56–65.

77. Blum Y, Belting HG, Ellertsdottir E, Herwig L, Luders F, et al. Complex cell rearrangements during intersegmental vessel sprouting and vessel fusion in the zebrafish embryo. Dev Biol. 2008;316:312–22.

78. Isogai S, Lawson ND, Torrealday S, Horiguchi M, Weinstein BM. Angiogenic network formation in the developing vertebrate trunk. Development. 2003;130:5281–90.
79. Fantin A, Vieira JM, Gestri G, Denti L, Schwarz Q, et al. Tissue macrophages act as cellular chaperones for vascular anastomosis downstream of VEGF-mediated endothelial tip cell induction. Blood. 2011;116:829–40.
80. Rymo SF, Gerhardt H, Wolfhagen Sand F, Lang R, Uv A, et al. A two-way communication between microglial cells and angiogenic sprouts regulates angiogenesis in aortic ring cultures. PLoS One. 2011;6, e15846.
81. Childs S, Chen JN, Garrity DM, Fishman MC. Patterning of angiogenesis in the zebrafish embryo. Development. 2002;129:973–82.
82. Carmeliet P, Tessier-Lavigne M. Common mechanisms of nerve and blood vessel wiring. Nature. 2005;436:193–200.
83. Gerhardt H, Golding M, Fruttiger M, Ruhrberg C, Lundkvist A, et al. VEGF guides angiogenic sprouting utilizing endothelial tip cell filopodia. J Cell Biol. 2003;161:1163–77.
84. Hellstrom M, Phng LK, Hofmann JJ, Wallgard E, Coultas L, et al. Dll4 signalling through Notch1 regulates formation of tip cells during angiogenesis. Nature. 2007;445:776–80.
85. Phng LK, Potente M, Leslie JD, Babbage J, Nyqvist D, et al. Nrarp coordinates endothelial Notch and Wnt signaling to control vessel density in angiogenesis. Dev Cell. 2009;16:70–82.
86. Jakobsson L, Franco CA, Bentley K, Collins RT, Ponsioen B, et al. Endothelial cells dynamically compete for the tip cell position during angiogenic sprouting. Nat Cell Biol. 2010;12:943–53.
87. Welsh AO, Enders AC. Chorioallantoic placenta formation in the rat: I. Luminal epithelial cell death and extracellular matrix modifications in the mesometrial region of implantation chambers. Am J Anat. 1991;192:215–31.
88. Welsh AO, Enders AC. Chorioallantoic placenta formation in the rat: II. Angiogenesis and maternal blood circulation in the mesometrial region of the implantation chamber prior to placenta formation. Am J Anat. 1991;192:347–65.
89. Kaloglu C, Gursoy E, Onarlioglu B. Early maternal changes contributing to the formation of the chorioallantoic and yolk sac placentas in rat: a morphological study. Anat Histol Embryol. 2003;32:200–6.
90. Osol G, Mandala M. Maternal uterine vascular remodeling during pregnancy. Physiology (Bethesda). 2009;24:58–71.
91. Brosens I, Robertson WB, Dixon HG. The physiological response of the vessels of the placental bed to normal pregnancy. J Pathol Bacteriol. 1967;93:569–79.
92. Lim HJ, Wang H. Uterine disorders and pregnancy complications: insights from mouse models. J Clin Invest. 2010;120:1004–15.
93. Ramathal CY, Bagchi IC, Taylor RN, Bagchi MK. Endometrial decidualization: of mice and men. Semin Reprod Med. 2010;28:17–26.
94. Matsumoto H, Ma WG, Daikoku T, Zhao X, Paria BC, et al. Cyclooxygenase-2 differentially directs uterine angiogenesis during implantation in mice. J Biol Chem. 2002;277:29260–7.
95. Douglas NC, Tang H, Gomez R, Pytowski B, Hicklin DJ, et al. Vascular endothelial growth factor receptor 2 (VEGFR-2) functions to promote uterine decidual angiogenesis during early pregnancy in the mouse. Endocrinology. 2009;150:3845–54.
96. Ma GT, Roth ME, Groskopf JC, Tsai FY, Orkin SH, et al. GATA-2 and GATA-3 regulate trophoblast-specific gene expression in vivo. Development. 1997;124:907–14.
97. Zhang J, Chen Z, Smith GN, Croy BA. Natural killer cell-triggered vascular transformation: maternal care before birth? Cell Mol Immunol. 2011;8:1–11.
98. Tanaka M, Gertsenstein M, Rossant J, Nagy A. Mash2 acts cell autonomously in mouse spongiotrophoblast development. Dev Biol. 1997;190:55–65.
99. Rossant J, Cross JC. Placental development: lessons from mouse mutants. Nat Rev Genet. 2001;2:538–48.

100. Watson ED, Cross JC. Development of structures and transport functions in the mouse placenta. Physiology (Bethesda). 2005;20:180–93.
101. Tanaka S, Kunath T, Hadjantonakis AK, Nagy A, Rossant J. Promotion of trophoblast stem cell proliferation by FGF4. Science. 1998;282:2072–5.
102. Anson-Cartwright L, Dawson K, Holmyard D, Fisher SJ, Lazzarini RA, et al. The glial cells missing-1 protein is essential for branching morphogenesis in the chorioallantoic placenta. Nat Genet. 2000;25:311–4.
103. Simmons DG, Natale DR, Begay V, Hughes M, Leutz A, et al. Early patterning of the chorion leads to the trilaminar trophoblast cell structure in the placental labyrinth. Development. 2008;135:2083–91.
104. Simmons DG, Fortier AL, Cross JC. Diverse subtypes and developmental origins of trophoblast giant cells in the mouse placenta. Dev Biol. 2007;304:567–78.
105. Georgiades P, Ferguson-Smith AC, Burton GJ. Comparative developmental anatomy of the murine and human definitive placentae. Placenta. 2002;23:3–19.
106. Hu D, Cross JC. Development and function of trophoblast giant cells in the rodent placenta. Int J Dev Biol. 2010;54:341–54.
107. Brosens IA, Robertson WB, Dixon HG. The role of the spiral arteries in the pathogenesis of pre-eclampsia. J Pathol. 1970;101:Pvi.
108. Brosens I, Pijnenborg R, Vercruysse L, Romero R. The "Great Obstetrical Syndromes" are associated with disorders of deep placentation. Am J Obstet Gynecol. 2010;204:193–201.
109. Zhou Y, Damsky CH, Fisher SJ. Preeclampsia is associated with failure of human cytotrophoblasts to mimic a vascular adhesion phenotype. One cause of defective endovascular invasion in this syndrome? J Clin Invest. 1997;99:2152–64.
110. Zhou Y, Fisher SJ, Janatpour M, Genbacev O, Dejana E, et al. Human cytotrophoblasts adopt a vascular phenotype as they differentiate. A strategy for successful endovascular invasion? J Clin Invest. 1997;99:2139–51.
111. Aharon A, Brenner B, Katz T, Miyagi Y, Lanir N. Tissue factor and tissue factor pathway inhibitor levels in trophoblast cells: implications for placental hemostasis. Thromb Haemost. 2004;92:776–86.
112. Lanir N, Aharon A, Brenner B. Procoagulant and anticoagulant mechanisms in human placenta. Semin Thromb Hemost. 2003;29:175–84.
113. Sood R, Kalloway S, Mast AE, Hillard CJ, Weiler H. Fetomaternal cross talk in the placental vascular bed: control of coagulation by trophoblast cells. Blood. 2006;107:3173–80.
114. Cross JC, Hemberger M, Lu Y, Nozaki T, Whiteley K, et al. Trophoblast functions, angiogenesis and remodeling of the maternal vasculature in the placenta. Mol Cell Endocrinol. 2002;187:207–12.
115. Screen M, Dean W, Cross JC, Hemberger M. Cathepsin proteases have distinct roles in trophoblast function and vascular remodelling. Development. 2008;135:3311–20.
116. Jackson D, Volpert OV, Bouck N, Linzer DI. Stimulation and inhibition of angiogenesis by placental proliferin and proliferin-related protein. Science. 1994;266:1581–4.
117. He Y, Smith SK, Day KA, Clark DE, Licence DR, et al. Alternative splicing of vascular endothelial growth factor (VEGF)-R1 (FLT-1) pre-mRNA is important for the regulation of VEGF activity. Mol Endocrinol. 1999;13:537–45.
118. Clark DE, Smith SK, He Y, Day KA, Licence DR, et al. A vascular endothelial growth factor antagonist is produced by the human placenta and released into the maternal circulation. Biol Reprod. 1998;59:1540–8.
119. Basyuk E, Cross JC, Corbin J, Nakayama H, Hunter P, et al. Murine Gcm1 gene is expressed in a subset of placental trophoblast cells. Dev Dyn. 1999;214:303–11.
120. Demir R, Kayisli UA, Seval Y, Celik-Ozenci C, Korgun ET, et al. Sequential expression of VEGF and its receptors in human placental villi during very early pregnancy: differences between placental vasculogenesis and angiogenesis. Placenta. 2004;25:560–72.
121. Coultas L, Chawengsaksophak K, Rossant J. Endothelial cells and VEGF in vascular development. Nature. 2005;438:937–45.

122. Ciruna BG, Schwartz L, Harpal K, Yamaguchi TP, Rossant J. Chimeric analysis of fibroblast growth factor receptor-1 (Fgfr1) function: a role for FGFR1 in morphogenetic movement through the primitive streak. Development. 1997;124:2829–41.
123. Dumont DJ, Fong GH, Puri MC, Gradwohl G, Alitalo K, et al. Vascularization of the mouse embryo: a study of flk-1, tek, tie, and vascular endothelial growth factor expression during development. Dev Dyn. 1995;203:80–92.
124. Yamaguchi TP, Harpal K, Henkemeyer M, Rossant J. fgfr-1 is required for embryonic growth and mesodermal patterning during mouse gastrulation. Genes Dev. 1994;8:3032–44.
125. Hirashima M, Lu Y, Byers L, Rossant J. Trophoblast expression of fms-like tyrosine kinase 1 is not required for the establishment of the maternal-fetal interface in the mouse placenta. Proc Natl Acad Sci U S A. 2003;100:15637–42.
126. Ema M, Takahashi S, Rossant J. Deletion of the selection cassette, but not cis-acting elements, in targeted Flk1-lacZ allele reveals Flk1 expression in multipotent mesodermal progenitors. Blood. 2006;107:111–7.
127. Sakurai Y, Ohgimoto K, Kataoka Y, Yoshida N, Shibuya M. Essential role of Flk-1 (VEGF receptor 2) tyrosine residue 1173 in vasculogenesis in mice. Proc Natl Acad Sci U S A. 2005;102:1076–81.
128. Deng CX, Wynshaw-Boris A, Shen MM, Daugherty C, Ornitz DM, et al. Murine FGFR-1 is required for early postimplantation growth and axial organization. Genes Dev. 1994;8:3045–57.
129. Carmeliet P, Moons L, Luttun A, Vincenti V, Compernolle V, et al. Synergism between vascular endothelial growth factor and placental growth factor contributes to angiogenesis and plasma extravasation in pathological conditions. Nat Med. 2001;7:575–83.
130. Autiero M, Waltenberger J, Communi D, Kranz A, Moons L, et al. Role of PlGF in the intra- and intermolecular cross talk between the VEGF receptors Flt1 and Flk1. Nat Med. 2003;9:936–43.
131. Carlstrom M, Wentzel P, Skott O, Persson AE, Eriksson UJ. Angiogenesis inhibition causes hypertension and placental dysfunction in a rat model of preeclampsia. J Hypertens. 2009;27:829–37.
132. Rutland CS, Mukhopadhyay M, Underwood S, Clyde N, Mayhew TM, et al. Induction of intrauterine growth restriction by reducing placental vascular growth with the angioinhibin TNP-470. Biol Reprod. 2005;73:1164–73.
133. Maynard SE, Min JY, Merchan J, Lim KH, Li J, et al. Excess placental soluble fms-like tyrosine kinase 1 (sFlt1) may contribute to endothelial dysfunction, hypertension, and proteinuria in preeclampsia. J Clin Invest. 2003;111:649–58.
134. Venkatesha S, Toporsian M, Lam C, Hanai J, Mammoto T, et al. Soluble endoglin contributes to the pathogenesis of preeclampsia. Nat Med. 2006;12:642–9.
135. Purwosunu Y, Sekizawa A, Yoshimura S, Farina A, Wibowo N, et al. Expression of angiogenesis-related genes in the cellular component of the blood of preeclamptic women. Reprod Sci. 2009;16:857–64.
136. Vaisbuch E, Whitty JE, Hassan SS, Romero R, Kusanovic JP, et al. Circulating angiogenic and antiangiogenic factors in women with eclampsia. Am J Obstet Gynecol. 2011;204:152. e1–9.
137. Wang A, Rana S, Karumanchi SA. Preeclampsia: the role of angiogenic factors in its pathogenesis. Physiology (Bethesda). 2009;24:147–58.
138. Reynolds LP, Borowicz PP, Caton JS, Vonnahme KA, Luther JS, et al. Uteroplacental vascular development and placental function: an update. Int J Dev Biol. 2010;54:355–66.
139. North PE, Waner M, Mizeracki A, Mrak RE, Nicholas R, et al. A unique microvascular phenotype shared by juvenile hemangiomas and human placenta. Arch Dermatol. 2001;137:559–70.
140. North PE, Waner M, Buckmiller L, James CA, Mihm Jr MC. Vascular tumors of infancy and childhood: beyond capillary hemangioma. Cardiovasc Pathol. 2006;15:303–17.

141. Frieden IJ, Haggstrom AN, Drolet BA, Mancini AJ, Friedlander SF, et al. Infantile hemangiomas: current knowledge, future directions. Proceedings of a research workshop on infantile hemangiomas, April 7–9, 2005, Bethesda, Maryland, USA. Pediatr Dermatol. 2005;22:383–406.
142. Barnes CM, Huang S, Kaipainen A, Sanoudou D, Chen EJ, et al. Evidence by molecular profiling for a placental origin of infantile hemangioma. Proc Natl Acad Sci U S A. 2005;102:19097–102.
143. North PE, Waner M, Brodsky MC. Are infantile hemangioma of placental origin? Ophthalmology. 2002;109:223–4.
144. Brouillard P, Vikkula M. Genetic causes of vascular malformations. Hum Mol Genet. 2007;16 Spec No. 2:R140–9.
145. Boon LM, Mulliken JB, Vikkula M, Watkins H, Seidman J, et al. Assignment of a locus for dominantly inherited venous malformations to chromosome 9p. Hum Mol Genet. 1994;3:1583–7.
146. Filston HC. Hemangiomas, cystic hygromas, and teratomas of the head and neck. Semin Pediatr Surg. 1994;3:147–59.
147. Werner JA, Dunne AA, Folz BJ, Rochels R, Bien S, et al. Current concepts in the classification, diagnosis and treatment of hemangiomas and vascular malformations of the head and neck. Eur Arch Otorhinolaryngol. 2001;258:141–9.
148. Boon LM, Brouillard P, Irrthum A, Karttunen L, Warman ML, et al. A gene for inherited cutaneous venous anomalies ("glomangiomas") localizes to chromosome 1p21-22. Am J Hum Genet. 1999;65:125–33.
149. Brouillard P, Boon LM, Mulliken JB, Enjolras O, Ghassibe M, et al. Mutations in a novel factor, glomulin, are responsible for glomuvenous malformations ("glomangiomas"). Am J Hum Genet. 2002;70:866–74.
150. Wang QK. Update on the molecular genetics of vascular anomalies. Lymphat Res Biol. 2005;3:226–33.
151. Pramanik K, Chun CZ, Garnaas MK, Samant GV, Li K, et al. Dusp-5 and Snrk-1 coordinately function during vascular development and disease. Blood. 2009;113:1184–91.
152. van der Putte SC. The early development of the lymphatic system in mouse embryos. Acta Morphol Neerl Scand. 1975;13:245–86.
153. Fong GH, Zhang L, Bryce DM, Peng J. Increased hemangioblast commitment, not vascular disorganization, is the primary defect in flt-1 knock-out mice. Development. 1999;126:3015–25.
154. Boivin B, Zhang S, Arbiser JL, Zhang ZY, Tonks NK. A modified cysteinyl-labeling assay reveals reversible oxidation of protein tyrosine phosphatases in angiomyolipoma cells. Proc Natl Acad Sci U S A. 2008;105:9959–64.
155. Perry BN, Govindarajan B, Bhandarkar SS, Knaus UG, Valo M, et al. Pharmacologic blockade of angiopoietin-2 is efficacious against model hemangiomas in mice. J Invest Dermatol. 2006;126:2316–22.

Chapter 4
The Genetic Basis and Molecular Diagnosis of Vascular Tumors and Developmental Malformations

Monte S. Willis and Tara Sander

Vascular Malformations

Vascular malformations, unlike vascular tumors, are present at birth (although not always evident), grow in proportion with the child, and do not regress. Although benign, they often present extremely challenging, lifelong management problems for patient and physician. Vascular malformations are defined by the affected vessel(s) and include capillary, venous, arterial, lymphatic, and combined malformations. Some are deadly, while others merely cosmetically or functionally disabling. Most are sporadic in occurrence, but more rare familial forms have revealed genetic abnormalities that not only suggest eventual therapies but also reveal basic control points in vasculogenesis (Table 4.1) [1–4].

Capillary Malformations (CMs)

Capillary malformations are slow-flow vascular malformations present at birth that grow with an individual, do not regress on their own, and have a normal rate of endothelial cell turnover. These contrast to infantile capillary hemangiomas

M.S. Willis, MD, PhD (✉)
Pathology & Laboratory Medicine; McAllister Heart Institute, University of North Carolina/
UNC Hospitals, 111 Mason Farm Road, 2340B MBRB, NC 27599 Chapel Hill, USA
e-mail: monte_willis@med.unc.edu

T. Sander, PhD
Department of Pathology and Laboratory Medicine, Children's Hospital of Wisconsin,
9000 W. Wisconsin Ave, Milwaukee, WI 53226, USA

Department of Pathology, Division of Pediatric Pathology, Medical College of Wisconsin,
8701 Watertown Plank Rd., Milwaukee, WI 53226, USA
e-mail: sandert@mcw.edu

© Springer Science+Business Media New York 2016
P.E. North, T. Sander (eds.), *Vascular Tumors and Developmental Malformations*,
Molecular and Translational Medicine, DOI 10.1007/978-1-4939-3240-5_4

Table 4.1 Molecular diagnostic targets and associations of vascular tumors and developmental malformations [1–4]

Vascular anomaly	Gene/locus	Location	Inheritance
Capillary/venulocapillary malformation			
Sturge-Weber syndrome (leptomeningeal and cutaneous venulocapillary malformation, aka "port-wine stain")	*GNAQ	9q21	Somatic
Non-syndromic port-wine stain	*GNAQ	9q21	Somatic
Arteriovenous malformations			
Capillary malformation-arteriovenous malformation (CM-AVM)	*RASA1	5q14.3	AD
Parkes Weber syndrome	*RASA1 (in subset)	5q14.3	AD
Hereditary hemorrhagic telangiectasia			
HHT1	*ENG	9q34.11	AD
HHT2	*ACVRL1/ALK1	12q13.13	AD
HHT3	Unknown	5q31.3-q32	AD
HHT4	Unknown	7p14	AD
Juvenile polyposis/HHT syndrome (JP/HHT)	*SMAD4	18q21.2	AD
HHT5/atypical HTT	*BMP9/GDF2	10q11.22	AD
HBT	Unknown	CMC1/5q14	Association only
Angiokeratoma			
Fabry disease	*GLA	Xq22.1	XD
Progressive patchy capillary malformations			
Angioma serpiginosum	Unknown	Xp11.3-Xq12	Association only
Familial cerebral cavernous malformations (CCM)			
CCM1	*KRIT1	7q21.2	AD
CCM2	*Malcavernin/CCM2	7p13	AD
CCM3	*PDCD10	3q26.1	AD
CCM4	Unknown	3q26.3-27.2	AD

Venous malformations

Sporadic Venous malformations (VM)	*TEK/TIE2	9p21.2	Somatic
Familial venous malformations cutaneous-mucosal (VMCM)	*TEK/TIE2	9p21.2	AD
Glomuvenous malformation (GVM)	*Glomulin/GLMN	1p22.1	AD
Verrucous venous malformation (VVM)/verrucous hemangioma	MAP3K3	17q23.3	Somatic

Lymphatic malformations, lymphedemas, and complex syndromes

CLOVES	*PIK3CA	3q26.32	Somatic
Klippel-Trenaunay syndrome (KTS)	*PIK3CA	3q26.32	Somatic
Fibro-adipose vascular anomaly (FAVA)	*PIK3CA	3q26.32	Somatic
Macrocephaly-capillary malformation (M-CM)	*PIK3CA	3q26.32	Somatic
Microcephaly-capillary malformation (MICCAP)	*STAMBP	2p13.1	AR
Nonne-Milroy syndrome	*FLT4/VEGFR3	5q34-35	AD/AR
Primary hereditary lymphedema (Nonne-Milroy-like syndrome)	*VEGFC	4q34	AD
Hypotrichosis lymphedema telangiectasia (HLT)	*SOX18	20q13.33	AD/AR
Primary hereditary lymphedema	*GJC2/Connexin 47	1q41-42, 4q34	AD
Lymphedema distichiasis	*FOXC2	16q24.1	AD
Primary lymphedema with myelodysplasia (Emberger syndrome)	*GATA2	3q21.3	AD
Primary generalized lymphatic anomaly (Hennekam syndrome)	*CCBE1	18q21.32	AR
Microcephaly with or without chorioretinopathy, lymphedema, or mental retardation syndrome	*KIF11	10q23.33	AD
Lymphedema-choanal atresia	*PTPN14	1q41	AR
Proteus syndrome	*AKT1	14q32.33	Somatic

(continued)

Table 4.1 (continued)

Vascular anomaly	Gene/locus	Location	Inheritance
Vascular tumors			
Infantile hemangioma	Unknown	5q31-33	Association only
Epithelioid hemangioendothelioma (EHE)	WWTR1-CAMTA1, YAP1-TFE3	t(1;3)(p36.23;q25.1), t(11;X)(q13;p11)	
Spindle cell hemangioma (Maffucci syndrome)	*IDH1, *IDH2	2q34, 15q26.1	Somatic
PTEN hamartoma tumor syndrome (PHTS)			
Bannayan-Riley-Ruvalcaba syndrome (BRRS)	*PTEN	10q23.3	AD
Cowden syndrome (CS)/Cowden-like syndrome	*PTEN, *SDHB, *SDHD, KLLN	10q23.3	AD
"Proteus-like" syndrome	*PTEN	10q23.3	AD
PTEN-related Proteus syndrome (PS)	*PTEN	10q23.3	AD

AD autosomal dominant, *AR* autosomal recessive, *XD* X-linked dominant

*Clinical testing available in the United States and/or internationally as of June 1, 2015, according to the GTR: Genetic Testing Registry at NCBI and www.GeneTests.org

which are highly proliferative, appear after birth, and have a characteristic rapid growth, slow involution, and marked cellular increase in endothelial cells [5, 6]. Capillary malformations occur in approximately 0.3 % of newborns in the United States and in 0.1–2 % of newborns worldwide [7]. Isolated capillary malformations do not increase mortality; however, they do cause disability secondary to facial disfigurement. One study has shown that psychosocial difficulties not only persist into adulthood, they actually get worse [8]. The most common capillary malformation is called a "port-wine stain" (aka nevus flammeus, OMIM 163000), resulting from a congenital malformation of the superficial vessels of the dermis, which is present at birth. Sturge-Weber syndrome is characterized by a port-wine stain of the face combined with capillary-venous malformations in the eye and brain (leptomeningeal angioma) [9]. Port-wine stains and Sturge-Weber syndrome are caused by a somatic mutation in the guanine nucleotide binding protein (GNAQ) on chromosome 9q21 [10]. A single-nucleotide variant in GNAQ (c.548G>A, p.Arg183Gln) was identified in 88 % of affected tissue samples from individuals with Sturge-Weber syndrome and 92 % from nonsyndromic port-wine stains [10]. Port-wine stains generally grow in proportion to the child and do not tend to involute spontaneously. Histologically, these vessels are lined by flat, endothelial cells, similar to the vessels found in the skin. They stain for endothelial antigens such as von Willebrand factor and collagenous basement membrane proteins. There are a paucity of mitotic cells similar to normal dermal vessels, indicating their turnover is not increased. They are found in the reticular dermis, with a mean depth of 0.46 mm [11]. There are both sporadic and familial forms that occur (Table 4.1).

Arteriovenous Malformations

Mutations in RASA1 Result in CM-AVM, AVF, and Parkes Weber Syndrome

Distinct from the nevus flammeus lesion is the autosomal dominant fast-flow capillary malformation-arteriovenous malformation (CM-AVM) characterized by AVM's and small, multifocal cutaneous vascular marks that may have a surrounding pale halo [12, 13]. Three distinct pathologies have been defined, all resulting from RASA1 mutations: (1) capillary malformation-arteriovenous malformation (CM-AVM, OMIM 608354), (2) arteriovenous fistula (AVF), and (3) Parkes Weber syndrome (PSW, OMIM 608355). Recent studies have found that these lesions result from loss-of-function mutations in the RASA1 gene [14]. Mutations in RASA1 would be present in a number of cell types, resulting in alterations in proliferation, migration, and survival, including endothelial cells that largely make up the malformation. The RASA1 gene encodes a protein that stimulates the GTPase activity of RAS p21, controlling cellular proliferation and differentiation. Mutations causing CM-AVM have a high penetrance, nearly 98 % [13]. Nearly 30 % of the time, CM-AVM lesions have associated vascular anomalies that are clinically more serious, including fast-flow anomalies like arteriovenous malformation (AVM), arteriovenous fistulas (AVF), or Parkes Weber syndrome (PWS) [13]. Eighty percent of the AVM and AVF are found in the head and neck regions [13]. For these reasons, a brain MRI is performed on patients presenting with CM-AVM found anywhere on the body. The heterogeneity of this disease process may be due to the requirement of additional somatic genetic hits or second mutations acquired [15]. Diagnosis of these three syndromes is made by sequencing the RASA1 gene, which is performed by a number of laboratories (Table 4.1).

Hereditary Hemorrhagic Telangiectasia

Hereditary hemorrhagic telangiectasia (HHT) or Rendu-Osler-Weber syndrome is an autosomal dominant disorder characterized by telangiectases and arteriovenous malformation (AVM) (OMIM 187300 and 600736) [16]. Several genes in the TGF-b/BMP signaling pathway are involved in hereditary hemorrhagic telangiectasia, including the genes endoglin (ENG), activin A receptor type II-like 1 (ACVRL1/ALK1), and SMAD4 [17]. Genetic variations in ENG, ACVRL1/ALK1, and SMAD4 cause HHT1, HHT2, and the combined juvenile polyposis/HHT (JP/HHT) syndrome, respectively (Table 4.1) [18–20]. Two additional loci, 5q31 and 7p14, are associated with HHT3 and HHT4, but the genes are unknown [21, 22]. Most of the disease-causing mutations identified in ENG, ACVRL1/ALK1, and SMAD4 are null alleles, resulting in haploinsufficiency and reduced protein levels in patients suffering from hereditary hemorrhagic telangiectasia [17]. Germline mutations are most common, but de novo mutations and mosaicism in ENG and ACVRL1/ALK1 have been reported [23]. In a few cases of telangiectases with atypical distribution, mutations in the bone morphogenetic 9 (BMP9) gene (GDF2) were identified [24]. In addition, genetic variants in PTPN14 and ADAM17 appear to be genetic modifiers of hereditary hemorrhagic telangiectasia that influence clinical severity [25, 26]. Molecular diagnostic testing is available for detection of mutations, large deletions, and duplications in ENG, ACVRL1/ALK1, SMAD4, and GDF2/BMP9. Endoglin and ACVRL1/ALK1 mutations are present in the majority of cases with an indicated suspicion of HHT, whereas SMAD is detected in less than 2 % of cases [17]. BMP9/GDF2 mutations appear to be rare, in less than 1 % of hereditary hemorrhagic telangiectasia. As such, ENG and ACVRL1/ALK1 are often tested first, simultaneously, with reflex to SMAD testing if results are negative for both genes [17].

Hereditary benign telangiectasias (HBT) are considered the benign form of hereditary hemorrhagic telangiectasia, characterized by asymptomatic lesions that can cause mild cosmetic disability [27]. HBT has been mapped to the CMC1 locus on chromosome 5q14 [27], although subsequent studies suggest that this phenotype may have other genetic causes as well [28].

Angiokeratoma

Angiokeratomas are capillary vascular malformations that are characterized as papules or plaques. These benign cutaneous lesions appear as small raised nodules that are red to blue and can be quite dark. A systemic form of angiokeratomas, known as angiokeratoma corporis diffusum, has been linked to metabolic disorders such as Fabry disease and fucosidosis and is transmitted in an autosomal dominant pattern (OMIM ID 60041). In the description of the systemic disease, skin lesions could be as limited to a few localized angiokeratomas on the scrotum, to more than 100 lesions over the limbs and trunk [29]. Single solitary lesions have also been reported on the tongue and oral cavity [30, 31]. Fabry disease is caused by genetic variations in alpha-galactosidase (GLA). Over 300 mutations have been identified in GLA, as well as several GLA gene rearrangements and mRNA processing defects [3]. Genetic testing is available to confirm diagnosis of a metabolic storage disorder, such as Fabry disease, in an individual with clinical and biochemical phenotype.

Progressive Patchy Capillary Malformations and Focal Dermal Hypoplasia

Progressive patchy capillary malformations (aka angioma serpiginosum) are a rare X-linked dominant congenital disorder [32]. It is characterized by increased numbers of dilated, thickened capillaries located sub-epidermally [32]. These findings are associated with mild hair and nail dystrophy and esophageal papillomas [32]. Affected individuals have a 112 kilobase deletion at Xp11.23 loci, which contains up to eight genes [33] (summarized in Table 4.1). However, genetic testing for progressive patch capillary malformation/angioma serpiginosum specifically is not currently available since the genetic basis has not been confirmed. A previously unrelated disorder, called focal dermal hypoplasia (FDH), is caused only by sporadic or inherited mutations and deletions in the PORCN gene, one of the genes located in the Xp11.23 loci missing in progressive patchy capillary malformations. FDH manifests itself as dermal atrophy, cutaneous and esophageal papillomas, as well as hand, eye, and skeletal anomalies [33–35]. While genetic testing for progressive patch capillary malformations does not exist, genetic testing for candidate genes, specifically PORCN, FTSJ1, and EBP, is available. However, not enough is currently understood about the genetics causing this disease to currently warrant use of these tests.

Familial Cerebral Cavernous Malformations (CCMs)

Cerebral cavernous malformations are familial vascular malformations [36] characterized by clustered capillary caverns within a single endothelium layer without normal brain parenchyma or mature vessel wall elements interrupting. The diameter of these vessels can vary from just a couple of millimeters to several cm. The cavern (channel) size and number progressively increase over time. The lesions themselves may develop de novo as demonstrated by serial MRIs and brain biopsies, demonstrating the evolutionary nature of CCMs [37].

CCMs occur in 0.4–0.5 % of the general population and are responsible for 5–15 % of all vascular malformation found in the cerebral cortex [36, 38, 39]. While CCM is found in children, the majority of patients do not have symptoms until they are adults. Patients generally present at a mean age of 30–40, with women presenting more commonly with hemorrhage and neurologic deficits [38, 39]. Up to 25 % remain symptom-free their entire life [40, 41], although other investigators have suggested this is an underestimation. Otten et al. [42], for example, reported an absence of symptoms in 90 % of CCMs identified at autopsy. The remaining 50–75 % present with a variety of symptoms, including cerebral hemorrhage, headaches, focal neurologic defects, and seizures [39]. CCM can be considered familial if these defects are seen in at least two family members or there are disease-causing mutations that are identified in genes associated with CCM. In cases without a family history, sporadic mutations are believed to account for the disease.

Clinical Diagnosis

The diagnosis of CCM is made by identifying blood flow through cavernous malformations. Not all malformations may be seen by angiography, making other modalities, such as MRI, more important in diagnosis [36]. T1 and T2 weighted images will show a characteristic popcorn pattern of variable intensities. On T2 or gradient echo, a dark hemosiderin ring at the periphery of the lesion may be seen, suggestive of a previous hemorrhage. Histopathologic examination and molecular testing are also utilized in making the diagnosis of CCM. Histologically, CCMs are identified by vascular malformations consisting of clustered, enlarged channels with a single layer of endothelium without intervening mature vessel wall elements or brain parenchyma [43–45].

Molecular Diagnosis of CCM

Familial CCM is associated with mutations in KRIT1, CCM2, and PDCD10 (Table 4.1), which account for 60–80 % of patients with CCM [46–49]. A putative locus for CCM has been proposed by Liquori et al. to be in the 3q26.3-27.2 region, although the specific gene involved has not been identified [48]. A single mutation in the KRIT1 gene, C1363T, is a common mutation found in 70 % of affected families of Hispanic heritage [50–52]. No other common mutation has been identified in other subgroups.

Molecular Pathogenesis of CCM

CCM1/KRIT1

CCM1 is caused by mutations in the gene KRIT1, located on 7q11.2-q21. The gene is comprised of 16 exons. Seventy four mutations have been described: 50 % are frameshifts, 24 % involve invariant splice junction changes, 24 % nonsense mutations, and 1 involves a deletion [53–56]. These mutations are distributed from exons 9 to 18 and are hypothesized to have a loss-of-function phenotype, since most result in a premature termination codon [55, 56]. The KRIT1 protein has tumor suppressor function and plays a critical role in early angiogenesis and the formation of vessels [57]. Mice lacking CCM1 are embryonic lethal, apparently due to its effects on the vasculature, more than its support for neurons [58].

CCM2/Malcavernin

The CCM2 gene product is the protein malcavernin, composed of 10 coding exons that encode a scaffold protein that functions in the p38 MAPK signaling cascade. Malcavernin interacts with the SMAD specific E3 ubiquitin ligase (SMURF1) through binding via a phosphotyrosine-binding domain to promote RhoA degradation [59]. Malcavernin is integral to normal cytoskeletal structure, cell-cell interactions, and formation of the lumen by endothelial cells [60].

CCM3/PDCD10

The PDCD10 (programmed cell death protein 10) gene has 10 exons, with the coding region starting in exon 4. This gene is an evolutionarily conserved protein that interacts with the serine/threonine protein kinase MST4 to regulate the ERK pathway [61]. At least seven mutations have been described in eight families, including a deletion of the entire gene and abnormal splicing of exon 5, three nonsense mutations, and two splice-site mutations [46]. Recent studies have implicated PDCD10 in cardiovascular development, in part by stabilizing the VEGF receptor [62–64] and by its role in apoptosis [65].

Molecular Testing for CCM

Clinical testing of KRIT1, CCM2, and PDCD10 is available (Table 4.1). In non-Hispanic individuals with a positive family history or multiple CCMs, KRIT1 mutations could be found in 43 % of probands with at least one affected relative or multiple CCM lesions detected by MRI [53]. Mutations in KRIT1 were identified in 30 % of individuals with multiple CCMs with no family history [66]. Thirteen to 20 % of patients with familial CCM have mutations in the CCM2 gene [54, 55, 67, 68]. In individuals with no family history of CCM, no Malcavernin/CCM2 mutations were found in one report [66]. While initial studies suggested 40 % of patients with familial CCM may be linked to PDCD10 [55, 67], more recent studies suggest this might be an overestimate. In patients with no mutation in KRIT1 or Malcavernin/CCM2 by sequence analysis, PDCD10 sequence analysis found between 7 % and 40 % [46–49]. Since 20–40 % of individuals from families with CCM do not have mutations in KRIT1, Malcavernin/CCM2, or PDCD10, linkage analysis to the CCM4 locus may be warranted [48]. However, this is done on a research testing basis only.

Genetic Counseling

Since familial CCM is autosomal dominant, identifying CCM mutations necessitates investigation of both parents and siblings. Many patients diagnosed with CCM have an asymptomatic parent. Alternatively, an affected proband may have CCM resulting from a de novo gene mutation. How often this occurs has not been studied thoroughly, as only one de novo germline mutation has been reported [69]. Caution should be taken when there is a negative family history because of the failure to recognize the disorder (asymptomatic), a reduced penetrance in the parent with a disease-causing mutation, and the possibility of an early death of an affected family member. Screening of parents may be performed by MRI [70].

The risk to the siblings of a proband depends on the presence of mutations in the proband's parents. If a proband's parent has a mutation, there is a 50 % risk to the siblings of inheriting the mutation. Offspring of a proband also has a 50 % risk of inheriting the mutations. If a parent is found to have a disease-causing mutation, it is recommended that family members be tested. If a mutation is not detected in the parents, the risk to the sibling is low as germline mosaicism has not been reported. In this case, it is likely that the proband has a de novo mutation, although alternate possibilities such as an undisclosed parent may be possible as well. Prenatal testing and preimplantation diagnosis are available for pregnancies at increased risk or for family planning (Table 4.1).

Venous Malformations

Venous anomalies are slow-flow lesions characterized by abnormal vascular channels lined by flat but continuous endothelial cells and smooth muscle cells that can be immature and deficient in number [71]. Venous anomalies are categorized into sporadic venous malformation (VM), familial venous malformations-multiple cutaneous or mucosal (VMCM), and glomuvenous malformation (GVM). VM, VMCM, and GVM are clinically distinguishable with regard to physical appearance, histology, genetic analysis, and management [71–74]. VM and VMCM are associated with gain-of-function mutations in receptor *TIE2*, whereas GVM is caused by loss-of-function mutations in the *glomulin* gene. These molecular signatures have allowed physicians to more accurately diagnose vascular anomalies and offer better managed treatment and care.

Sporadic Venous Malformation (VM) and Familial Cutaneous and Mucosal Venous Malformation (VMCM)

Most venous malformations (94 %) are sporadic vascular malformations (VMs) with unifocal (93 %) or multifocal (1 %) presentation. VMs are light to dark blue lesions that are compressible on palpation [72, 74]. They grow proportionally with the child and can be more invasive to the muscles, tissues, and organs [74].

Inherited VMCMs (MIM# 600195; Orpha.net #2451) are hereditary vascular malformations often characterized by small, multifocal lesions that have a bluish purple color [72]. VMCMs account for approximately 1 % of all vascular anomalies. VMCMs are also known as venous malformations-multiple cutaneous and mucosal, cutaneomucosal, and mucocutaneous venous malformations. VMCMs demonstrate autosomal dominant inheritance with incomplete penetrance. Therefore, each child of an affected individual will have a 50 % risk of inheriting the disease-causing mutation.

TIE2 Mutations in VM and VMCM

To date, receptor tyrosine kinase *TIE2* (also known as TEK) is the only gene known to be associated with VM and VMCM. *TIE2* is a receptor tyrosine kinase almost exclusively expressed in vascular endothelial cells (OMIM 600221). The *TIE2* gene maps to human locus 9p21 and consists of 23 exons that span over 121 kb of the genome. *TIE2* has a well-documented role in embryonic development, primarily through the binding of the growth factor ligand angiopoietin-1 (ANG1), which triggers downstream signaling pathways required for angiogenesis and vasculogenesis.

Mutations in *TIE2* have been identified in familial and sporadic VMCM cases. The most common mutation is the arginine to tryptophan substitution at position 849 (R849W) in the kinase domain of *TIE2*, with an incidence of 60 % [72]. The R849W *TIE2* mutation was identified by segregation in two different families with dominantly inherited vascular malformation [75]. Subsequent studies confirmed the R849W mutation and identified seven additional *TIE2* germline mutations in different families (Y897S, Y897C, R915H, R918C, V919L, A925S, K1100N) [76–78].

Eight somatic "second hit" alterations have also been found in lesions from individuals with multiple sporadic VM [79]. Six of these mutations are novel (Y897H, Y897F, L914F, R915C, R915L, S917I), while two were previously identified in the germline of patients with VMCM (Y897S and Y897C) [76, 78]. The most common somatic mutation, L914F, is found alone and accounts for 85 % of lesions [72]. The other lesions contain pairs of double mutations in *cis* [72]. The identification of a second somatic mutation in the lesion suggests a paradominant mode of inheritance. Similar to R849W, all *TIE2* mutations are located in the tyrosine kinase domains of the receptor and result in ligand-dependent hyperphosphorylation [72, 78]. In vivo and in vitro studies demonstrate increased *TIE2* activity and ligand-dependent hyperphosphorylation in several mutations, including R849W [75, 76, 78, 79]. Thus, *TIE2* mutations associated with VMCM render a gain-of-function phenotype.

Molecular Genetic Testing

Clinical testing of the *TIE2* gene is available [80] (Table 4.1). Methods include mutation scanning and sequence analysis of variants. In certain cases, prenatal diagnosis may be available for affected families in which a disease-causing mutation has been identified [80]. Germline mutations in VMCM are identified by analysis of genomic DNA isolated from whole blood specimens of individuals with VMCM. To identify the presence of a second somatic mutation specific to the VMCM disorder, genetic analysis of the lesion is important for accurate diagnosis.

Glomuvenous Malformation (GVM)

GVMs are hereditary vascular malformations characterized by small, multifocal lesions with a cobblestone-like appearance that have a pink to purplish dark blue color [71, 72, 81] (MIM #138000; Orpha.net #83454). A venous malformation containing round mural "glomus cells" is diagnosed as a GVM. GVMs account for approximately 5 % of all vascular anomalies [72, 74]. GVMs are also known as venous malformations with glomus cells (VMGLOM), glomangiomatosis, familial or hereditary glomangiomas, and glomus tumors of the skin and soft tissue.

Glomulin Mutations in GVM

Glomulin (also known as *GLMN* and *FAP68*) is the only gene known to date that is associated with GVM. In two separate studies, 7 of 12 families with inherited GVM showed linkage to a region of 1.48 Mbp in the VMGLOM locus on chromosome 1p22-p21 [82, 83]. Positional cloning then identified *glomulin* as the gene within the VMGLOM locus that was responsible for GVMs [84, 85]. The *glomulin* gene consists of 19 exons spanning over 55 kb of the genome and encodes a 594-amino acid protein (also known as FAP68). Previous studies had cloned the incomplete *glomulin* cDNA sequence encoding a predicted 417-amino acid protein of 48 kDa, which is also known as FKBP-associated protein (FAP48) [86].

GVMs demonstrate an autosomal dominant mode of inheritance with incomplete penetrance. Accordingly, the child of an affected individual has a 50 % chance of inheriting the germline mutation. Current evidence supports the hypothesis that all GVMs are caused by loss-of-function mutations in the *glomulin* gene [73, 81]. More than 30 different *glomulin* mutations have been identified in >100 GVM families [81, 87–90]. Eight glomulin mutations are common (i.e., 108C > A, 157delAAGAA, 554delA + 556delCCT, and 1179delCAA) and found in >75 % of patients with GVM [88]. There also appears to be a strong founder effect [72, 81]. In a small percentage of patients, a second somatic mutation in *glomulin* (*in trans*) is also seen in combination with the inherited (germline) *glomulin* mutation, suggesting a paradominant mode of inheritance. The remaining mutations have been identified in only one GVM family to date [81]. It appears that all *glomulin* mutations result in truncated glomulin protein, except for one (1179delCCA), which results in a deletion of an arginine at position 394 [81].

Neither in vitro nor in vivo studies have been performed to demonstrate the specific type of functional loss for *glomulin* or definitively determine specific genotype-phenotype associations. This is because the function of *glomulin* remains poorly understood. Furthermore, clinical correlations between specific *glomulin* mutations and the location, extent, and number of vascular lesions have not been made [91]. It is known that glomulin is predominantly expressed in vascular smooth muscle cells (VSMCs) [92]. Glomus cells of GVMs are histologically characterized as abnormally differentiated VSMCs [93], suggesting *glomulin* is involved in VSMC differentiation and its functional loss results in the immature glomus cell phenotype seen in GVM [84].

Molecular Genetic Testing

Clinical testing for GVMs via mutation screening of the GLVM gene is available (Table 4.1). Platforms include analysis of the entire coding region by sequencing and analysis of the entire coding region by mutation scanning. Germline mutations in *glomulin* are identified by analysis of genomic DNA isolated from whole blood specimens. Analysis of genomic DNA from resected tissue is important to identify the presence of a second somatic mutation specific to the GVM lesion. At least one laboratory offers prenatal diagnosis for a known *glomulin* mutation.

Lymphatic Malformations and Lymphedemas

Lymphatic malformations (LM) are focal or extensive lesions of dilated lymphatic channels with abnormal connection to the lymphatic system [88]. They are a major component feature in patients with congenital lipomatous overgrowth with vascular, epidermal, and skeletal anomaly (CLOVES) syndrome and Klippel-Trenaunay syndrome (KTS). Lymphatic malformations occur sporadically, suggesting the presence of somatic mutations. Recently, five somatic mutations in phosphatidylinositol-4,5-biphosphate 3-kinase, catalytic subunit alpha (PIK3CA) have been identified in patients with lymphatic malformations, CLOVES, KTS, and fibroadipose vascular anomaly (FAVA) [94, 95].

Lymphedemas are characterized by a defect in lymphatic drainage, which results in accumulation of lymphatic fluid in the interstitial space and severe swelling of the lower extremities [72, 88]. Lymphedemas can be sporadic or inherited as an incompletely penetrant autosomal dominant trait or recessive form (see Table 4.1). Studies in families with inherited forms of lymphedema have identified several genes causing the disorders. Nonne-Milroy syndrome is an early onset, primary congenital form of hereditary type I lymphedema that is autosomal dominantly inherited. Loss-of-function mutations in *FLT4/VEGFR3* at chromosome location 5q34-35 are associated with autosomal dominant Nonne-Milroy syndrome, as well as recessively inherited lymphedemas [96, 97]. A mutation in VEGFC, a ligand for VEGFR3, has also been identified in a family with clinical signs resembling Nonne-Milroy syndrome [4]. Lymphedema distichiasis is a syndromic form of primary lymphedema, which is an autosomal dominant disease caused by loss-of-function mutations in *FOXC2* located on chromosome 16p24 [98]. Hypotrichosis lymphedema telangiectasia (HLT) syndrome is inherited as a recessive or dominant trait. Nonsense and homozygous mutations in *SOX18* on chromosome 20q13.33 are responsible for the HLT disorder [99]. More recently, GJC2 (encoding connexin 47) missense mutations were also observed to cause primary lymphedema [100]. The genetic cause and/or locus has been identified for other more rare forms of familial lymphedema. These include *CCBE1* on chromosome 18q21.32, *NEMO* on chromosome Xq28, genetic locus 6q16.2-q22.1, and chromosome 15q, which are associated with Hennekam syndrome, OLEDAID, primary congenital resolving lymphedema, and hereditary lymphedema cholestasis (HLC), respectively (Aagenaes syndrome) (Table 4.1) [101–104]. PTPN14, GATA2, and KIF11 germline mutations are also associated with lymphedemas in choanal atresia, Emberger syndrome, and microcephaly chorioretinopathy, respectively [2].

Vascular Tumors

Vascular tumors are cellular, often proliferative vascular anomalies including infantile hemangiomas (IHs), congenital hemangiomas (RICH and NICH), kaposiform hemangioendotheliomas, tufted angioma, spindle cell hemangioendotheliomas, as well as other rare hemangioendotheliomas and dermatologic acquired vascular tumors [105]. Infantile hemangiomas are the most common tumors of infancy, affecting approximately 4 % of all children and are far more common than vascular malformations. There are also several clinical subtypes and syndromes associated with IHs. An example is PHACE(S) syndrome (posterior fossa malformations, hemangiomas, arterial anomalies, coarctation of the aorta and cardiac defects, eye abnormalities and sterna defects), which involves facial IHs in association with other anomalies [106, 107]. Hemangiomatosis, PELVIS syndrome, and SACRAL syndrome are other examples [105].

Infantile hemangiomas (OMIM #602089) are comprised of rapidly proliferating endothelial cells that typically appear shortly after birth, grow rapidly during the first year, and then slowly involute over a period of several years. Although all infantile hemangiomas spontaneously regress to a significant degree, most leave clinically significant sequelae, and some are life-threatening. Clinically useful therapeutic options include systemic or local corticosteroids, surgical excision, laser therapy, vincristine, immunomodulatory therapy, and most recently, treatment with beta-blockers such as propranolol. Mechanisms of most medical therapies are largely unknown, and no therapies are universally successful. Recent advances in understanding basic pathogenetic mechanisms yield hope for more effective, specifically targeted therapies.

Diagnosis of Vascular Tumors

Most vascular tumors are differentially diagnosed by their presentation, growth pattern, histological profile, and use of MRI to determine the density and high-flow patterns [105]. Infantile hemangiomas are characterized by strong endothelial GLUT-1 protein expression, which is not seen in other vascular tumors or in normal skin vasculature [108].

The genetics of infantile hemangiomas is poorly understood, although linkage analysis and microarray and cellular studies have identified several important pathogenetic features and candidate genes that may contribute to predilection for the disease. Genome-wide linkage analysis of three unrelated cases of infantile hemangioma led to the identification of a disease locus on chromosome 5q31-33 containing candidate genes FGFGR4, PDGFR-β, and VEGFR3 (Flt-4) [109]. In addition, somatic mutations in the genes VEGFR2 (P1147S), VEGFR3/FLT4 (P954S), TEM8, and DUSP5 genes have been identified in hemangioma tumor tissue [109]. The link between these mutations and disease is not established. It has been hypothesized that germline mutations in TEM8 and KDR represent risk factor mutations for IH and that the combination of these mutations with a secondary somatic hit may trigger the expansion of hemangioma-derived endothelial cells within the lesions [105].

More recent discoveries have been made for other vascular anomalies. For example, a somatic missense mutation (c.1323C>G, p. Iso441Met) in mitogen-activated protein kinase kinase kinase 3 (MAP3K3) has been identified in verrucous venous malformations (verrucous hemangioma) [110]. In addition, the presence of YAP1-TFE3 and WWTR1-CAMTA1 gene fusions has been reported in subsets of epithelioid hemangioendothelioma (EHE) [111, 112], which is a rare malignant soft tissue tumor of variable grade [113].

Somatic mutations in IDH1 or IDH2 have been identified in patients with Maffucci syndrome [114–118]. Maffucci syndrome is a rare congenital disorder characterized by multiple central cartilaginous tumors (enchondromas), similar to

Ollier disease, but with multiple cutaneous spindle cell hemangiomas (SCH) [115]. Common heterozygous point mutations include R132C and R132H in IDH1, as well as the R172S mutation in IDH2. Additional studies found that frequent somatic alterations in 2p22.3, 2q24.3, and 14q11.2 may play a role in causing enchondroma and SCH in patients with Maffucci syndrome [115]. Clinical testing is available for IDH1 and IDH2.

Pharmacogenetics and Treatment of Vascular Anomalies

Managed treatment of vascular anomalies often involves drug therapy, which can cause mild to severe adverse side effects. For example, propranolol is a nonselective beta-adrenergic blocker commonly used to treat cardiac disorders that has gained recent attention in the vascular anomaly community for its off-label use in the treatment of infantile hemangiomas [119–124]. An initial improvement in the size and color of the hemangiomas is observed and the effect is proposed to be secondary to the factors that affect angiogenesis. However, there are known side effects in some patients treated with propranolol, including hypoglycemia, hypothermia, and bradycardia [125].

Pharmacogenetics uses an individual's genotype to help predict drug response, efficacy, and potential adverse drug events. As such, pharmacogenetics could be applied to the IH population during drug therapy. Propranolol is one of the drugs from the top 200 list eliminated by cytochrome P450 (CYP450) enzymes, which contain single-nucleotide polymorphisms (SNPs) that alter enzymatic function [126, 127]. For example, propranolol is metabolized by CYP2D6 and CYP1A2 and enzymes contain SNPs associated with decreased enzymatic activity [128, 129]. Genetic polymorphisms in the β1 and β2-adrenergic receptors, targets of propranolol, have also been identified that affect gene expression, protein function, and response to beta-agonists [130, 131]. Therefore, individuals with SNPs in metabolizing enzymes and/or receptor targets could have an altered drug response to therapy. Pharmacogenetic testing has the potential of offering a direct application to the vascular anomalies population for optimizing treatment and reducing side effects. However, while pharmacogenetic testing is available in several reference and hospital-based laboratories, application to the vascular anomaly population is new and requires additional studies.

PTEN Hamartoma Tumor Syndrome

We have included the PTEN hamartoma tumor syndrome (PHTS) because of the emerging understanding that vascular anomalies are a distinct and common finding in the spectrum of PHTS disease [132]. Vascular anomalies in patients with PTEN mutations typically manifest as multifocal intramuscular combinations of ectopic fat and fast-flow channels with cerebral developmental venous anomalies particularly common [132]. Arteriovenous malformations have been described in Cowden syndrome [133], which may be due to PTEN's regulation of vascular development and angiogenesis by directly regulating VEGF and other angiogenic factors [134]. So even though small abnormal tumors on the skin and in critical organs dominate the clinical diagnosis of PHTS spectrum diseases, vascular anomalies are a critical feature of this group of diseases.

PTHS is a group of disorders with mutation in the PTEN gene and includes (1) Cowden syndrome (CS), (2) Bannayan-Riley-Ruvalcaba syndrome (BRRS), (3) *PTEN*-related Proteus syndrome (PS), and (4) Proteus-like syndrome. All four of these diseases have in common the presence of hamartomas or abnormal formation of benign tissue "tumors." These "tumors" cause problems primarily due to their location, particularly when they are located on the face and neck, where they can cause significant disfigurement. While these abnormal growths can obstruct any organ in the body, they tend to cause the most health problems when they are located in the hypothalamus, spleen, or kidneys. PTHS must not be confused with Proteus syndrome, which is a rare complex disease characterized by disproportionate bony and soft tissue overgrowth caused by mutations in AKT1. AKT1 activity is regulated by PTEN, so both proteins are involved in intracellular PI3K/Akt signaling [3].

The diagnosis of PTEN hamartoma tumor syndrome (PHTS) is based on specific clinical findings. However, the diagnosis of PHTS is made only when a disease-causing mutation in PTEN is identified. Diagnostic criteria have been developed for Cowden syndrome [135, 136]. Diagnostic criteria for BRRS have not been developed, but are based largely on the cardinal feature of microcephaly, hamartomatous intestinal polyposis, lipomas, and glans penis pigmented macules [137]. *PTEN-related* Proteus syndrome (PS) is widely variable and generally has a mosaic distribution. The manifestations present generally at birth and include cystadenoma of the ovary, various types of testicular tumors, CNS tumor, and parotid monomorphic adenomas. Only 120 people with PS have been identified [138] and diagnostic criteria have been developed by Biesecker et al. [139]. While diagnostic criteria have not been developed for Proteus-like syndrome, it generally includes patients with features of Proteus syndrome, who do not meet the criteria [140].

The phosphatase and tensin homolog (PTEN) protein is a tumor suppressor protein encoded by the *PTEN* gene. PTEN is part of a subclass of phosphatases that have dual activities which remove phosphates from tyrosine as well as serine and threonine. PTEN is critical to the de-phosphorylation of phospho-inositide-3,4,5-triphosphate, resulting in a down-regulation of the downstream Akt signaling pathway. PTEN traffics in and out of the nucleus [141–143] and when in the nucleus inhibits MAPK signaling resulting in an arrest of the cell cycle [144, 145]. In the cytoplasm, PTEN's activity primarily stimulates Akt activity to induce apoptosis [146]. Germline mutations have been identified in exons 1–8 (of 9 total) and include missense, nonsense, splice-site mutations, insertions, and large deletions [147–149]. Approximately 40 % of mutations have been reported in exon 5 [136]; however, most mutations are unique, but recurrent mutations have been found [147–149].

Clinical molecular testing for disease-causing mutations in PTEN is most commonly performed by analysis of the entire coding region by sequencing (Table 4.1). Many laboratories also perform molecular analyses to identify deletions and duplications, which can be missed by sequencing. Currently, at least one laboratory focuses sequencing on select regions of the PTEN gene in addition to performing FISH-metaphase analysis of mutations (Table 4.1).

Sequence Analysis of PTEN

Nearly all of the missense mutations identified in PTEN are deleterious [136]. Nearly 85 % of patients who meet criteria for Cowden's syndrome and 65 % with a diagnosis of BRRS have a PTEN mutation [149–151]. PTEN mutations are found in 20 % of patients with Proteus syndrome and 50 % of those with a Proteus-like syndrome [136, 148, 152–154]. Another study found that no PTEN mutations could be identified in patients diagnosed with Proteus-like syndrome [155]. These studies suggest that either other genes are involved or else mutations in introns/splice sites or promoters were present and not detected using the methodologies applied. Additionally, deletion and duplications could have been present and not detected. On a research basis, direct sequencing of the promoter regions of PTEN can be performed, which alters the function of the PTEN gene product. Approximately 10 % of CS patients have promoter mutations and no other mutations identified in the coding region [151].

Identification of Deletions and Duplications in PTEN

Individuals with CS who have large deletions have been reported [156]. Additionally, up to 10 % of BRRS patients do not have a mutation that can be detected in the PTEN exons due to deletions within PTEN [151]. Real-time PCR, Southern blotting, Multiplex ligation-dependent probe amplification (MLPA), and other methods that can detect gene copy can be used to determine PTEN deletions or other rearrangements, which PCR-based sequencing is unable to detect.

Non-PTEN Gene Mutations Affecting Susceptibility to Disease

In addition to PTEN mutations, recent early studies have identified mutations in succinate dehydrogenase complex subunit B (SDHB) and succinate dehydrogenase complex subunit D (SDHD), the genes encoding the mitochondrial complex II protein succinate dehydrogenase, as well as the KLLN (killin) gene in individuals with CS and CS-like disorder [157, 158].

Testing Strategies

Ideally, sequence analysis of PTEN exons 1–9, including the flanking introns, is performed to confirm the diagnosis in a proband (see Table 4.1). Analysis of the PTEN promoter region can be performed next (on a research basis), followed by deletion and duplication analysis (see Table 4.1). Lastly, mutations in the mitochondrial complex II protein succinate dehydrogenase (SDH) have been described in PTEN mutation-negative individuals with CS-like cancers [157]. So sequence analysis of SDH may be warranted, which is available on a research basis for other diseases (testing for SHD B performed for hereditary paraganglioma-pheochromocytoma syndromes).

Differentiating Genetically Related Disorders

One of the challenges of genetically diagnosing Cowden syndrome (CS), Bannayan-Riley-Ruvalcaba syndrome (BRRS), *PTEN*-related Proteus syndrome (PS), and Proteus-like syndrome is that mutations in PTEN underlie other diseases with diametrically opposed phenotypes. No other phenotypes other than CS, BRRS, PS, and Proteus-like syndrome are consistently caused by PTEN mutations. Adult-onset Lhermitte-Duclos disease (LDD) can be attributed sometimes to PTEN mutations and characterized by dysplastic gangliocytoma of the cerebellum due to the overgrowth of hamartomas, which can be seen in CS/BRRS. However, PTEN mutations are rarely seen in the LDD form of disease, which presents in childhood [159]. Similarly, PTEN mutations have been reported in ~20 % of people with autism/pervasive developmental disorder and macrocephaly [160, 161]. Several groups have now confirmed this PTEN mutation in 10–20 % of people with autism/pervasive developmental disorder and macrocephaly [161–164].

Genetic Counseling

Patients with PTEN hamartoma tumor syndrome (PHTS) should be advised that the disease is autosomal dominant, so that testing of family members should be recommended. However, since disease is both sporadic and familial, some individuals with CS have no family history, with a rough estimate of 10–50 % having an affected parent [165]. If a proband has an identifiable PTEN mutation, their parents should undergo a clinical evaluation and be tested to identify if PHTS is present.

Testing of proband siblings depends on the genetic status of the parents. If a parent has a PTEN mutation, siblings should be tested since this is an autosomal dominant disease. If neither parent has a PTEN mutation that is identifiable, the proband siblings do not need to be tested. The risk of disease in proband siblings is minimal since mosaicism in the germline has not been reported in PHTS [140]. If the proband does not have an identifiable PTEN mutation, PHTS can be excluded by clinical evaluation of the sibling. Each offspring of a proband has a 50 % chance of inheriting the mutation and developing the PHTS. Therefore, genetic testing should be performed on all offspring of a proband. Prenatal testing is available from many laboratories (see Table 4.1).

Challenges and Future of Molecular Testing

Molecular Diagnostic Challenges

While the genetic cause for several inherited forms of vascular malformations is known, significant challenges facing the field include elucidating the etiology of sporadic forms, identifying somatic mutations that cause rare disorders, and developing therapies [88]. For example, TIE2 mutations account for 40–50 % of VMs, but additional mutations or predisposing genes responsible for the remaining cases are unknown [72]. Another problem is that the genotype-phenotype correlations are not well understood for many disorders, often because the function of the predisposing gene is not known (i.e., *glomulin* mutations associated with GVM). This hinders an understanding of the mechanism by which specific mutations cause disease and the discovery of therapeutic treatments. Finally, a major difficulty within the field is that molecular diagnostic testing for many vascular anomalies is not yet commercially available. Molecular tests that do currently exist are, in most cases, on a research basis only and many of these labs are located in European countries. Furthermore, insurance companies are not often willing to reimburse for genetic testing and turnaround times can be lengthy. This makes testing difficult, cumbersome, and costly for many families. The promising news for the field is that clinical laboratories can provide laboratory developed tests (LDTs) using standard, cost-effective technologies, such as sequencing, allele-specific PCR, and restriction enzymatic digestions [166]. Furthermore, high-density SNP arrays and next-generation sequencing provide the opportunity for high-throughput genotyping, which revolutionizes the way novel and known mutations associated with disease are identified and diagnosed. Advances in sequencing technology have led to a lower error rate, longer read length, and more robust performance, which far exceeds that of standard sequencing using Sanger methodology [167]. The application of next-generation sequencing to vascular disease has the potential to rapidly screen every gene in an affected individual and identify the mutation(s) associated with that particular vascular lesion. The laboratory is also able to identify novel mutations and provide more accurate diagnosis using technology that reduces tissue heterogeneity. Advances in automated extraction technology have allowed the lab to rapidly extract high-quality DNA from various pathology tissue specimens, both fresh/frozen and formalin-fixed paraffin-embedded (FFPE). Laser-capture microdissection also offers the capability of obtaining lesion-derived material and isolating a specific cell population for subsequent genotype analysis. Such analysis would require punch biopsy or surgical resection of the affected tissue. A limitation lies in the ability to isolate a sufficient number of cells for DNA, mRNA, or protein analysis. Cell culture expansion of isolated cell types is an alternative solution if an inadequate amount of tissue is not available for analysis. However, proper diagnosis based on mRNA on protein analysis will depend on the cells maintaining their phenotype once cultured.

References

1. ISSVA. Causal genes of vascular anomalies. In: ISSVA classification for vascular anomalies: approved at the 20th ISSVA workshop, Melbourne. 2014; pp. Appendix 2a–2f.
2. Blatt J, Powell CM, Burkhart CN, Stavas J, Aylsworth AS. Genetics of hemangiomas, vascular malformations, and primary lymphedema. J Pediatr Hematol Oncol. 2014;36:587–93.
3. Boon LM, Vikkula M. Molecular genetics of vascular malformations. In: Mulliken JB, Burrown PE, Fishman SJ, editors. Mulliken and Young's vascular anomalies: hemangiomas and malformations. Oxford: Oxford University Press; 2013.
4. Nguyen HL, Boon LM, Vikkula M. Genetics of vascular malformations. Semin Pediatr Surg. 2014;23:221–6.
5. Legiehn GM, Heran MK. Classification, diagnosis, and interventional radiologic management of vascular malformations. Orthop Clin North Am. 2006;37:435–74, vii–viii.
6. Spring MA, Bentz ML. Cutaneous vascular lesions. Clin Plast Surg. 2005;32:171–86.
7. Jacobs AH, Walton RG. The incidence of birthmarks in the neonate. Pediatrics. 1976; 58:218–22.
8. Lanigan SW, Cotterill JA. Psychological disabilities amongst patients with port wine stains. Br J Dermatol. 1989;121:209–15.
9. Comi AM. Presentation, diagnosis, pathophysiology, and treatment of the neurological features of Sturge-Weber syndrome. Neurologist. 2011;17:179–84.
10. Shirley MD, Tang H, Gallione CJ, Baugher JD, Frelin LP, Cohen B, North PE, Marchuk DA, Comi AM, Pevsner J. Sturge-Weber syndrome and port-wine stains caused by somatic mutation in GNAQ. N Engl J Med. 2013;368:1971–9.
11. Eubanks LE, McBurney EI. Videomicroscopy of port-wine stains: correlation of location and depth of lesion. J Am Acad Dermatol. 2001;44:948–51.
12. Boon LM, Mulliken JB, Vikkula M. RASA1: variable phenotype with capillary and arteriovenous malformations. Curr Opin Genet Dev. 2005;15:265–9.
13. Revencu N, Boon LM, Mulliken JB, Enjolras O, Cordisco MR, Burrows PE, Clapuyt P, Hammer F, Dubois J, Baselga E, et al. Parkes Weber syndrome, vein of Galen aneurysmal malformation, and other fast-flow vascular anomalies are caused by RASA1 mutations. Hum Mutat. 2008;29:959–65.
14. Eerola I, Boon LM, Mulliken JB, Burrows PE, Dompmartin A, Watanabe S, Vanwijck R, Vikkula M. Capillary malformation-arteriovenous malformation, a new clinical and genetic disorder caused by RASA1 mutations. Am J Hum Genet. 2003;73:1240–9.
15. Boon LM, Mulliken JB, Vikkula M, Watkins H, Seidman J, Olsen BR, Warman ML. Assignment of a locus for dominantly inherited venous malformations to chromosome 9p. Hum Mol Genet. 1994;3:1583–7.

16. Guttmacher AE, Marchuk DA, White Jr RI. Hereditary hemorrhagic telangiectasia. N Engl J Med. 1995;333:918–24.
17. McDonald J, Wooderchak-Donahue W, VanSant Webb C, Whitehead K, Stevenson DA, Bayrak-Toydemir P. Hereditary hemorrhagic telangiectasia: genetics and molecular diagnostics in a new era. Front Genet. 2015;6:1.
18. Gallione CJ, Richards JA, Letteboer TG, Rushlow D, Prigoda NL, Leedom TP, Ganguly A, Castells A, Ploos van Amstel JK, Westermann CJ, et al. SMAD4 mutations found in unselected HHT patients. J Med Genet. 2006;43:793–7.
19. Johnson DW, Berg JN, Baldwin MA, Gallione CJ, Marondel I, Yoon SJ, Stenzel TT, Speer M, Pericak-Vance MA, Diamond A, et al. Mutations in the activin receptor-like kinase 1 gene in hereditary haemorrhagic telangiectasia type 2. Nat Genet. 1996;13:189–95.
20. Shovlin CL, Hughes JM, Tuddenham EG, Temperley I, Perembelon YF, Scott J, Seidman CE, Seidman JG. A gene for hereditary haemorrhagic telangiectasia maps to chromosome 9q3. Nat Genet. 1994;6:205–9.
21. Bayrak-Toydemir P, McDonald J, Akarsu N, Toydemir RM, Calderon F, Tuncali T, Tang W, Miller F, Mao R. A fourth locus for hereditary hemorrhagic telangiectasia maps to chromosome 7. Am J Med Genet A. 2006;140:2155–62.
22. Cole SG, Begbie ME, Wallace GM, Shovlin CL. A new locus for hereditary haemorrhagic telangiectasia (HHT3) maps to chromosome 5. J Med Genet. 2005;42:577–82.
23. Best DH, Vaughn C, McDonald J, Damjanovich K, Runo JR, Chibuk JM, Bayrak-Toydemir P. Mosaic ACVRL1 and ENG mutations in hereditary haemorrhagic telangiectasia patients. J Med Genet. 2011;48:358–60.
24. Wooderchak-Donahue WL, McDonald J, O'Fallon B, Upton PD, Li W, Roman BL, Young S, Plant P, Fulop GT, Langa C, et al. BMP9 mutations cause a vascular-anomaly syndrome with phenotypic overlap with hereditary hemorrhagic telangiectasia. Am J Hum Genet. 2013;93:530–7.
25. Benzinou M, Clermont FF, Letteboer TG, Kim JH, Espejel S, Harradine KA, Arbelaez J, Luu MT, Roy R, Quigley D, et al. Mouse and human strategies identify PTPN14 as a modifier of angiogenesis and hereditary haemorrhagic telangiectasia. Nat Commun. 2012;3:616.
26. Kawasaki K, Freimuth J, Meyer DS, Lee MM, Tochimoto-Okamoto A, Benzinou M, Clermont FF, Wu G, Roy R, Letteboer TG, et al. Genetic variants of Adam17 differentially regulate TGFbeta signaling to modify vascular pathology in mice and humans. Proc Natl Acad Sci U S A. 2014;111:7723–8.
27. Brancati F, Valente EM, Tadini G, Caputo V, Di Benedetto A, Gelmetti C, Dallapiccola B. Autosomal dominant hereditary benign telangiectasia maps to the CMC1 locus for capillary malformation on chromosome 5q14. J Med Genet. 2003;40:849–53.
28. Molho-Pessach V, Agha Z, Libster D, Lerer I, Burger A, Jaber S, Abeliovich D, Zlotogorski A. Evidence for clinical and genetic heterogeneity in hereditary benign telangiectasia. J Am Acad Dermatol. 2007;57:814–8.
29. Calzavara-Pinton PG, Colombi M, Carlino A, Zane C, Gardella R, Clemente M, Facchetti F, Moro L, Zoppi N, Caimi L, et al. Angiokeratoma corporis diffusum and arteriovenous fistulas with dominant transmission in the absence of metabolic disorders. Arch Dermatol. 1995;131:57–62.
30. Fernandez-Acenero MJ, Rey Biel J, Renedo G. Solitary angiokeratoma of the tongue in adults. Rom J Morphol Embryol. 2010;51:771–3.
31. Ranjan N, Mahajan VK. Oral angiokeratomas: proposed clinical classification. Int J Dermatol. 2009;48:778–81.
32. Blinkenberg EO, Brendehaug A, Sandvik AK, Vatne O, Hennekam RC, Houge G. Angioma serpiginosum with oesophageal papillomatosis is an X-linked dominant condition that maps to Xp11.3-Xq12. Eur J Hum Genet. 2007;15:543–7.
33. Houge G, Oeffner F, Grzeschik KH. An Xp11.23 deletion containing PORCN may also cause angioma serpiginosum, a cosmetic skin disease associated with extreme skewing of X-inactivation. Eur J Hum Genet. 2008;16:1027–8.

34. Grzeschik KH, Bornholdt D, Oeffner F, Konig A, del Carmen Boente M, Enders H, Fritz B, Hertl M, Grasshoff U, Hofling K, et al. Deficiency of PORCN, a regulator of Wnt signaling, is associated with focal dermal hypoplasia. Nat Genet. 2007;39:833–5.
35. Wang X, Reid Sutton V, Omar Peraza-Llanes J, Yu Z, Rosetta R, Kou YC, Eble TN, Patel A, Thaller C, Fang P, et al. Mutations in X-linked PORCN, a putative regulator of Wnt signaling, cause focal dermal hypoplasia. Nat Genet. 2007;39:836–8.
36. Rigamonti D, Hadley MN, Drayer BP, Johnson PC, Hoenig-Rigamonti K, Knight JT, Spetzler RF. Cerebral cavernous malformations. Incidence and familial occurrence. N Engl J Med. 1988;319:343–7.
37. Fritschi JA, Reulen HJ, Spetzler RF, Zabramski JM. Cavernous malformations of the brain stem. A review of 139 cases. Acta Neurochir (Wien). 1994;130:35–46.
38. Del Curling Jr O, Kelly Jr DL, Elster AD, Craven TE. An analysis of the natural history of cavernous angiomas. J Neurosurg. 1991;75:702–8.
39. Robinson JR, Awad IA, Little JR. Natural history of the cavernous angioma. J Neurosurg. 1991;75:709–14.
40. Siegel AM. Familial cavernous angioma: an unknown, known disease. Acta Neurol Scand. 1998;98:369–71.
41. Siegel AM, Andermann E, Badhwar A, Rouleau GA, Wolford GL, Andermann F, Hess K. Anticipation in familial cavernous angioma: a study of 52 families from International Familial Cavernous Angioma Study. IFCAS Group. Lancet. 1998;352:1676–7.
42. Otten P, Pizzolato GP, Rilliet B, Berney J. 131 cases of cavernous angioma (cavernomas) of the CNS, discovered by retrospective analysis of 24,535 autopsies. Neurochirurgie. 1989;35:82–3, 128–131.
43. Brunereau L, Levy C, Laberge S, Houtteville J, Labauge P. De novo lesions in familial form of cerebral cavernous malformations: clinical and MR features in 29 non-Hispanic families. Surg Neurol. 2000;53:475–82, discussion 482–473.
44. Rigamonti D, Drayer BP, Johnson PC, Hadley MN, Zabramski J, Spetzler RF. The MRI appearance of cavernous malformations (angiomas). J Neurosurg. 1987;67:518–24.
45. Zabramski JM, Wascher TM, Spetzler RF, Johnson B, Golfinos J, Drayer BP, Brown B, Rigamonti D, Brown G. The natural history of familial cavernous malformations: results of an ongoing study. J Neurosurg. 1994;80:422–32.
46. Bergametti F, Denier C, Labauge P, Arnoult M, Boetto S, Clanet M, Coubes P, Echenne B, Ibrahim R, Irthum B, et al. Mutations within the programmed cell death 10 gene cause cerebral cavernous malformations. Am J Hum Genet. 2005;76:42–51.
47. Guclu B, Ozturk AK, Pricola KL, Bilguvar K, Shin D, O'Roak BJ, Gunel M. Mutations in apoptosis-related gene, PDCD10, cause cerebral cavernous malformation 3. Neurosurgery. 2005;57:1008–13.
48. Liquori CL, Berg MJ, Squitieri F, Ottenbacher M, Sorlie M, Leedom TP, Cannella M, Maglione V, Ptacek L, Johnson EW, et al. Low frequency of PDCD10 mutations in a panel of CCM3 probands: potential for a fourth CCM locus. Hum Mutat. 2006;27:118.
49. Verlaan DJ, Roussel J, Laurent SB, Elger CE, Siegel AM, Rouleau GA. CCM3 mutations are uncommon in cerebral cavernous malformations. Neurology. 2005;65:1982–3.
50. Gunel M, Awad IA, Finberg K, Anson JA, Steinberg GK, Batjer HH, Kopitnik TA, Morrison L, Giannotta SL, Nelson-Williams C, et al. A founder mutation as a cause of cerebral cavernous malformation in Hispanic Americans. N Engl J Med. 1996;334:946–51.
51. Johnson EW, Iyer LM, Rich SS, Orr HT, Gil-Nagel A, Kurth JH, Zabramski JM, Marchuk DA, Weissenbach J, Clericuzio CL, et al. Refined localization of the cerebral cavernous malformation gene (CCM1) to a 4-cM interval of chromosome 7q contained in a well-defined YAC contig. Genome Res. 1995;5:368–80.
52. Sahoo T, Johnson EW, Thomas JW, Kuehl PM, Jones TL, Dokken CG, Touchman JW, Gallione CJ, Lee-Lin SQ, Kosofsky B, et al. Mutations in the gene encoding KRIT1, a Krev-1/rap1a binding protein, cause cerebral cavernous malformations (CCM1). Hum Mol Genet. 1999;8:2325–33.

53. Cave-Riant F, Denier C, Labauge P, Cecillon M, Maciazek J, Joutel A, Laberge-Le Couteulx S, Tournier-Lasserve E. Spectrum and expression analysis of KRIT1 mutations in 121 consecutive and unrelated patients with Cerebral Cavernous Malformations. Eur J Hum Genet. 2002;10:733–40.

54. Denier C, Goutagny S, Labauge P, Krivosic V, Arnoult M, Cousin A, Benabid AL, Comoy J, Frerebeau P, Gilbert B, et al. Mutations within the MGC4607 gene cause cerebral cavernous malformations. Am J Hum Genet. 2004;74:326–37.

55. Verlaan DJ, Davenport WJ, Stefan H, Sure U, Siegel AM, Rouleau GA. Cerebral cavernous malformations: mutations in Krit1. Neurology. 2002;58:853–7.

56. Verlaan DJ, Siegel AM, Rouleau GA. Krit1 missense mutations lead to splicing errors in cerebral cavernous malformation. Am J Hum Genet. 2002;70:1564–7.

57. Guzeloglu-Kayisli O, Amankulor NM, Voorhees J, Luleci G, Lifton RP, Gunel M. KRIT1/cerebral cavernous malformation 1 protein localizes to vascular endothelium, astrocytes, and pyramidal cells of the adult human cerebral cortex. Neurosurgery. 2004;54:943–9, discussion 949.

58. Whitehead KJ, Plummer NW, Adams JA, Marchuk DA, Li DY. Ccm1 is required for arterial morphogenesis: implications for the etiology of human cavernous malformations. Development. 2004;131:1437–48.

59. Crose LE, Hilder TL, Sciaky N, Johnson GL. Cerebral cavernous malformation 2 protein promotes smad ubiquitin regulatory factor 1-mediated RhoA degradation in endothelial cells. J Biol Chem. 2009;284:13301–5.

60. Stockton RA, Shenkar R, Awad IA, Ginsberg MH. Cerebral cavernous malformations proteins inhibit Rho kinase to stabilize vascular integrity. J Exp Med. 2010;207:881–96.

61. Ma X, Zhao H, Shan J, Long F, Chen Y, Zhang Y, Han X, Ma D. PDCD10 interacts with Ste20-related kinase MST4 to promote cell growth and transformation via modulation of the ERK pathway. Mol Biol Cell. 2007;18:1965–78.

62. He Y, Zhang H, Yu L, Gunel M, Boggon TJ, Chen H, Min W. Stabilization of VEGFR2 signaling by cerebral cavernous malformation 3 is critical for vascular development. Sci Signal. 2010;3:ra26.

63. Tanriover G, Seval Y, Sati L, Gunel M, Demir N. CCM2 and CCM3 proteins contribute to vasculogenesis and angiogenesis in human placenta. Histol Histopathol. 2009;24:1287–94.

64. Zheng X, Xu C, Di Lorenzo A, Kleaveland B, Zou Z, Seiler C, Chen M, Cheng L, Xiao J, He J, et al. CCM3 signaling through sterile 20-like kinases plays an essential role during zebrafish cardiovascular development and cerebral cavernous malformations. J Clin Invest. 2010;120:2795–804.

65. Lauenborg B, Kopp K, Krejsgaard T, Eriksen KW, Geisler C, Dabelsteen S, Gniadecki R, Zhang Q, Wasik MA, Woetmann A, et al. Programmed cell death-10 enhances proliferation and protects malignant T cells from apoptosis. APMIS. 2010;118:719–28.

66. Verlaan DJ, Laurent SB, Sure U, Bertalanffy H, Andermann E, Andermann F, Rouleau GA, Siegel AM. CCM1 mutation screen of sporadic cases with cerebral cavernous malformations. Neurology. 2004;62:1213–5.

67. Craig HD, Gunel M, Cepeda O, Johnson EW, Ptacek L, Steinberg GK, Ogilvy CS, Berg MJ, Crawford SC, Scott RM, et al. Multilocus linkage identifies two new loci for a mendelian form of stroke, cerebral cavernous malformation, at 7p15-13 and 3q25.2-27. Hum Mol Genet. 1998;7:1851–8.

68. Liquori CL, Berg MJ, Siegel AM, Huang E, Zawistowski JS, Stoffer T, Verlaan D, Balogun F, Hughes L, Leedom TP, et al. Mutations in a gene encoding a novel protein containing a phosphotyrosine-binding domain cause type 2 cerebral cavernous malformations. Am J Hum Genet. 2003;73:1459–64.

69. Lucas M, Costa AF, Montori M, Solano F, Zayas MD, Izquierdo G. Germline mutations in the CCM1 gene, encoding Krit1, cause cerebral cavernous malformations. Ann Neurol. 2001;49:529–32.

70. Johnson EW. Cerebral cavernous malformation, familial. In: Pagon RA, Bird TC, Dolan CR, Stephens K, editors. GeneReviews. Seattle: University of Washington; 2006.

71. Boon LM, Mulliken JB, Enjolras O, Vikkula M. Glomuvenous malformation (glomangioma) and venous malformation: distinct clinicopathologic and genetic entities. Arch Dermatol. 2004;140:971–6.
72. Boon LM, Ballieux F, Vikkula M. Pathogenesis of vascular anomalies. Clin Plast Surg. 2011;38:7–19.
73. Boon LM, Vikkula M. From blue jeans to blue genes. J Craniofac Surg. 2009;20 Suppl 1:703–6.
74. Dompmartin A, Vikkula M, Boon LM. Venous malformation: update on aetiopathogenesis, diagnosis and management. Phlebology. 2010;25:224–35.
75. Vikkula M, Boon LM, Carraway 3rd KL, Calvert JT, Diamonti AJ, Goumnerov B, Pasyk KA, Marchuk DA, Warman ML, Cantley LC, et al. Vascular dysmorphogenesis caused by an activating mutation in the receptor tyrosine kinase TIE2. Cell. 1996;87:1181–90.
76. Calvert JT, Riney TJ, Kontos CD, Cha EH, Prieto VG, Shea CR, Berg JN, Nevin NC, Simpson SA, Pasyk KA, et al. Allelic and locus heterogeneity in inherited venous malformations. Hum Mol Genet. 1999;8:1279–89.
77. Nobuhara Y, Onoda N, Fukai K, Hosomi N, Ishii M, Wakasa K, Nishihara T, Ishikawa T, Hirakawa K. TIE2 gain-of-function mutation in a patient with pancreatic lymphangioma associated with blue rubber-bleb nevus syndrome: report of a case. Surg Today. 2006;36:283–6.
78. Wouters V, Limaye N, Uebelhoer M, Irrthum A, Boon LM, Mulliken JB, Enjolras O, Baselga E, Berg J, Dompmartin A, et al. Hereditary cutaneomucosal venous malformations are caused by TIE2 mutations with widely variable hyper-phosphorylating effects. Eur J Hum Genet. 2010;18:414–20.
79. Limaye N, Wouters V, Uebelhoer M, Tuominen M, Wirkkala R, Mulliken JB, Eklund L, Boon LM, Vikkula M. Somatic mutations in angiopoietin receptor gene TEK cause solitary and multiple sporadic venous malformations. Nat Genet. 2009;41:118–24.
80. Boon LM, Vikkula M. Multiple cutaneous and mucosal venous malformations. In: GeneReviews – NCBI bookshelf [Internet]. Seattle: University of Washington; 2008.
81. Brouillard P, Ghassibe M, Penington A, Boon LM, Dompmartin A, Temple IK, Cordisco M, Adams D, Piette F, Harper JI, et al. Four common glomulin mutations cause two thirds of glomuvenous malformations ("familial glomangiomas"): evidence for a founder effect. J Med Genet. 2005;42, e13.
82. Boon LM, Brouillard P, Irrthum A, Karttunen L, Warman ML, Rudolph R, Mulliken JB, Olsen BR, Vikkula M. A gene for inherited cutaneous venous anomalies ("glomangiomas") localizes to chromosome 1p21-22. Am J Hum Genet. 1999;65:125–33.
83. Irrthum A, Brouillard P, Enjolras O, Gibbs NF, Eichenfield LF, Olsen BR, Mulliken JB, Boon LM, Vikkula M. Linkage disequilibrium narrows locus for venous malformation with glomus cells (VMGLOM) to a single 1.48 Mbp YAC. Eur J Hum Genet. 2001;9:34–8.
84. Brouillard P, Boon LM, Mulliken JB, Enjolras O, Ghassibe M, Warman ML, Tan OT, Olsen BR, Vikkula M. Mutations in a novel factor, glomulin, are responsible for glomuvenous malformations ("glomangiomas"). Am J Hum Genet. 2002;70:866–74.
85. Brouillard P, Olsen BR, Vikkula M. High-resolution physical and transcript map of the locus for venous malformations with glomus cells (VMGLOM) on chromosome 1p21-p22. Genomics. 2000;67:96–101.
86. Chambraud B, Radanyi C, Camonis JH, Shazand K, Rajkowski K, Baulieu EE. FAP48, a new protein that forms specific complexes with both immunophilins FKBP59 and FKBP12. Prevention by the immunosuppressant drugs FK506 and rapamycin. J Biol Chem. 1996;271:32923–9.
87. Goujon E, Cordoro KM, Barat M, Rousseau T, Brouillard P, Vikkula M, Frieden IJ, Vabres P. Congenital plaque-type glomuvenous malformations associated with fetal pleural effusion and ascites. Pediatr Dermatol. 2010;28:528–31.
88. Limaye N, Boon LM, Vikkula M. From germline towards somatic mutations in the pathophysiology of vascular anomalies. Hum Mol Genet. 2009;18:R65–74.
89. O'Hagan AH, Moloney FJ, Buckley C, Bingham EA, Walsh MY, McKenna KE, McGibbon D, Hughes AE. Mutation analysis in Irish families with glomuvenous malformations. Br J Dermatol. 2006;154:450–2.

90. Ostberg A, Moreno G, Su T, Trisnowati N, Marchuk D, Murrell DF. Genetic analysis of a family with hereditary glomuvenous malformations. Australas J Dermatol. 2007;48:170–3.
91. Chen AY, Eide M, Shwayder T. Glomuvenous malformation in a boy with transposition of the great vessels: a case report and review of literature. Pediatr Dermatol. 2009;26:70–4.
92. McIntyre BA, Brouillard P, Aerts V, Gutierrez-Roelens I, Vikkula M. Glomulin is predominantly expressed in vascular smooth muscle cells in the embryonic and adult mouse. Gene Expr Patterns. 2004;4:351–8.
93. Kato N, Kumakiri M, Ohkawara A. Localized form of multiple glomus tumors: report of the first case showing partial involution. J Dermatol. 1990;17:423–8.
94. Kurek KC, Luks VL, Ayturk UM, Alomari AI, Fishman SJ, Spencer SA, Mulliken JB, Bowen ME, Yamamoto GL, Kozakewich HP, et al. Somatic mosaic activating mutations in PIK3CA cause CLOVES syndrome. Am J Hum Genet. 2012;90:1108–15.
95. Luks VL, Kamitaki N, Vivero MP, Uller W, Rab R, Bovee JV, Rialon KL, Guevara CJ, Alomari AI, Greene AK, et al. Lymphatic and other vascular malformative/overgrowth disorders are caused by somatic mutations in PIK3CA. J Pediatr. 2015;166(1048–1054):e1041–5.
96. Ghalamkarpour A, Holnthoner W, Saharinen P, Boon LM, Mulliken JB, Alitalo K, Vikkula M. Recessive primary congenital lymphoedema caused by a VEGFR3 mutation. J Med Genet. 2009;46:399–404.
97. Irrthum A, Karkkainen MJ, Devriendt K, Alitalo K, Vikkula M. Congenital hereditary lymphedema caused by a mutation that inactivates VEGFR3 tyrosine kinase. Am J Hum Genet. 2000;67:295–301.
98. Finegold DN, Kimak MA, Lawrence EC, Levinson KL, Cherniske EM, Pober BR, Dunlap JW, Ferrell RE. Truncating mutations in FOXC2 cause multiple lymphedema syndromes. Hum Mol Genet. 2001;10:1185–9.
99. Irrthum A, Devriendt K, Chitayat D, Matthijs G, Glade C, Steijlen PM, Fryns JP, Van Steensel MA, Vikkula M. Mutations in the transcription factor gene SOX18 underlie recessive and dominant forms of hypotrichosis-lymphedema-telangiectasia. Am J Hum Genet. 2003;72:1470–8.
100. Ferrell RE, Baty CJ, Kimak MA, Karlsson JM, Lawrence EC, Franke-Snyder M, Meriney SD, Feingold E, Finegold DN. GJC2 missense mutations cause human lymphedema. Am J Hum Genet. 2010;86:943–8.
101. Alders M, Hogan BM, Gjini E, Salehi F, Al-Gazali L, Hennekam EA, Holmberg EE, Mannens MM, Mulder MF, Offerhaus GJ, et al. Mutations in CCBE1 cause generalized lymph vessel dysplasia in humans. Nat Genet. 2009;41:1272–4.
102. Bull LN, Roche E, Song EJ, Pedersen J, Knisely AS, van Der Hagen CB, Eiklid K, Aagenaes O, Freimer NB. Mapping of the locus for cholestasis-lymphedema syndrome (Aagenaes syndrome) to a 6.6-cM interval on chromosome 15q. Am J Hum Genet. 2000;67:994–9.
103. Doffinger R, Smahi A, Bessia C, Geissmann F, Feinberg J, Durandy A, Bodemer C, Kenwrick S, Dupuis-Girod S, Blanche S, et al. X-linked anhidrotic ectodermal dysplasia with immunodeficiency is caused by impaired NF-kappaB signaling. Nat Genet. 2001;27:277–85.
104. Malik S, Grzeschik KH. Congenital, low penetrance lymphedema of lower limbs maps to chromosome 6q16.2-q22.1 in an inbred Pakistani family. Hum Genet. 2008;123:197–205.
105. Jinnin M, Ishihara T, Boye E, Olsen BR. Recent progress in studies of infantile hemangioma. J Dermatol. 2010;37:283–98.
106. Frieden IJ, Reese V, Cohen D. PHACE syndrome. The association of posterior fossa brain malformations, hemangiomas, arterial anomalies, coarctation of the aorta and cardiac defects, and eye abnormalities. Arch Dermatol. 1996;132:307–11.
107. Schwartz RA, Sidor MI, Musumeci ML, Lin RL, Micali G. Infantile haemangiomas: a challenge in paediatric dermatology. J Eur Acad Dermatol Venereol. 2010;24:631–8.
108. North PE, Waner M, Mizeracki A, Mihm Jr MC. GLUT1: a newly discovered immunohistochemical marker for juvenile hemangiomas. Hum Pathol. 2000;31:11–22.
109. Walter JW, North PE, Waner M, Mizeracki A, Blei F, Walker JW, Reinisch JF, Marchuk DA. Somatic mutation of vascular endothelial growth factor receptors in juvenile hemangioma. Genes Chromosom Cancer. 2002;33:295–303.

110. Couto JA, Vivero MP, Kozakewich HP, Taghinia AH, Mulliken JB, Warman ML, Greene AK. A somatic MAP3K3 mutation is associated with verrucous venous malformation. Am J Hum Genet. 2015;96:480–6.
111. Antonescu CR, Le Loarer F, Mosquera JM, Sboner A, Zhang L, Chen CL, Chen HW, Pathan N, Krausz T, Dickson BC, et al. Novel YAP1-TFE3 fusion defines a distinct subset of epithelioid hemangioendothelioma. Genes Chromosom Cancer. 2013;52:775–84.
112. Flucke U, Vogels RJ, de Saint Aubain Somerhausen N, Creytens DH, Riedl RG, van Gorp JM, Milne AN, Huysentruyt CJ, Verdijk MA, van Asseldonk MM, et al. Epithelioid Hemangioendothelioma: clinicopathologic, immunohistochemical, and molecular genetic analysis of 39 cases. Diagn Pathol. 2014;9:131.
113. Antonescu C. Malignant vascular tumors – an update. Mod Pathol. 2014;27 Suppl 1:S30–8.
114. Amary MF, Damato S, Halai D, Eskandarpour M, Berisha F, Bonar F, McCarthy S, Fantin VR, Straley KS, Lobo S, et al. Ollier disease and Maffucci syndrome are caused by somatic mosaic mutations of IDH1 and IDH2. Nat Genet. 2011;43:1262–5.
115. Amyere M, Dompmartin A, Wouters V, Enjolras O, Kaitila I, Docquier PL, Godfraind C, Mulliken JB, Boon LM, Vikkula M. Common somatic alterations identified in maffucci syndrome by molecular karyotyping. Mol Syndromol. 2014;5:259–67.
116. Couvineau A, Wouters V, Bertrand G, Rouyer C, Gerard B, Boon LM, Grandchamp B, Vikkula M, Silve C. PTHR1 mutations associated with Ollier disease result in receptor loss of function. Hum Mol Genet. 2008;17:2766–75.
117. Kurek KC, Pansuriya TC, van Ruler MA, van den Akker B, Luks VL, Verbeke SL, Kozakewich HP, Sciot R, Lev D, Lazar AJ, et al. R132C IDH1 mutations are found in spindle cell hemangiomas and not in other vascular tumors or malformations. Am J Pathol. 2013;182:1494–500.
118. Pansuriya TC, van Eijk R, d'Adamo P, van Ruler MA, Kuijjer ML, Oosting J, Cleton-Jansen AM, van Oosterwijk JG, Verbeke SL, Meijer D, et al. Somatic mosaic IDH1 and IDH2 mutations are associated with enchondroma and spindle cell hemangioma in Ollier disease and Maffucci syndrome. Nat Genet. 2011;43:1256–61.
119. Buckmiller LM, Munson PD, Dyamenahalli U, Dai Y, Richter GT. Propranolol for infantile hemangiomas: early experience at a tertiary vascular anomalies center. Laryngoscope. 2010;120:676–81.
120. Chik KK, Luk CK, Chan HB, Tan HY. Use of propranolol in infantile haemangioma among Chinese children. Hong Kong Med J. 2010;16:341–6.
121. Leaute-Labreze C, Dumas de la Roque E, Hubiche T, Boralevi F, Thambo JB, Taieb A. Propranolol for severe hemangiomas of infancy. N Engl J Med. 2008;358:2649–51.
122. Sans V, de la Roque ED, Berge J, Grenier N, Boralevi F, Mazereeuw-Hautier J, Lipsker D, Dupuis E, Ezzedine K, Vergnes P, et al. Propranolol for severe infantile hemangiomas: follow-up report. Pediatrics. 2009;124:e423–31.
123. Truong MT, Perkins JA, Messner AH, Chang KW. Propranolol for the treatment of airway hemangiomas: a case series and treatment algorithm. Int J Pediatr Otorhinolaryngol. 2010;74:1043–8.
124. Zimmermann AP, Wiegand S, Werner JA, Eivazi B. Propranolol therapy for infantile haemangiomas: review of the literature. Int J Pediatr Otorhinolaryngol. 2010;74:338–42.
125. Lawley LP, Siegfried E, Todd JL. Propranolol treatment for hemangioma of infancy: risks and recommendations. Pediatr Dermatol. 2009;26:610–4.
126. Daly AK. Pharmacogenetics and human genetic polymorphisms. Biochem J. 2010;429:435–49.
127. Zanger UM, Turpeinen M, Klein K, Schwab M. Functional pharmacogenetics/genomics of human cytochromes P450 involved in drug biotransformation. Anal Bioanal Chem. 2008;392:1093–108.
128. Johnson JA, Herring VL, Wolfe MS, Relling MV. CYP1A2 and CYP2D6 4-hydroxylate propranolol and both reactions exhibit racial differences. J Pharmacol Exp Ther. 2000;294:1099–105.

129. Walle T, Walle UK, Cowart TD, Conradi EC, Gaffney TE. Selective induction of propranolol metabolism by smoking: additional effects on renal clearance of metabolites. J Pharmacol Exp Ther. 1987;241:928–33.
130. Liggett SB. Pharmacogenomics of beta1-adrenergic receptor polymorphisms in heart failure. Heart Fail Clin. 2010;6:27–33.
131. Litonjua AA, Gong L, Duan QL, Shin J, Moore MJ, Weiss ST, Johnson JA, Klein TE, Altman RB. Very important pharmacogene summary ADRB2. Pharmacogenet Genomics. 2010; 20:64–9.
132. Tan WH, Baris HN, Burrows PE, Robson CD, Alomari AI, Mulliken JB, Fishman SJ, Irons MB. The spectrum of vascular anomalies in patients with PTEN mutations: implications for diagnosis and management. J Med Genet. 2007;44:594–602.
133. Turnbull MM, Humeniuk V, Stein B, Suthers GK. Arteriovenous malformations in Cowden syndrome. J Med Genet. 2005;42, e50.
134. Hamada K, Sasaki T, Koni PA, Natsui M, Kishimoto H, Sasaki J, Yajima N, Horie Y, Hasegawa G, Naito M, et al. The PTEN/PI3K pathway governs normal vascular development and tumor angiogenesis. Genes Dev. 2005;19:2054–65.
135. Eng C. Will the real Cowden syndrome please stand up: revised diagnostic criteria. J Med Genet. 2000;37:828–30.
136. Eng C. PTEN: one gene, many syndromes. Hum Mutat. 2003;22:183–98.
137. Gorlin RJ, Cohen Jr MM, Condon LM, Burke BA. Bannayan-Riley-Ruvalcaba syndrome. Am J Med Genet. 1992;44:307–14.
138. Cohen Jr MM. Overgrowth syndromes: an update. Adv Pediatr. 1999;46:441–91.
139. Biesecker LG, Happle R, Mulliken JB, Weksberg R, Graham Jr JM, Viljoen DL, Cohen Jr MM. Proteus syndrome: diagnostic criteria, differential diagnosis, and patient evaluation. Am J Med Genet. 1999;84:389–95.
140. Eng C. PTEN hamartoma tumor syndrome (PHTS). In: Pagon RA, Bird TC, Dolan CR, Stephens K, editors. GeneReviews [Internet]. Seattle: University of Washington; 2009.
141. Chung JH, Eng C. Nuclear-cytoplasmic partitioning of phosphatase and tensin homologue deleted on chromosome 10 (PTEN) differentially regulates the cell cycle and apoptosis. Cancer Res. 2005;65:8096–100.
142. Ginn-Pease ME, Eng C. Increased nuclear phosphatase and tensin homologue deleted on chromosome 10 is associated with G0-G1 in MCF-7 cells. Cancer Res. 2003;63:282–6.
143. Minaguchi T, Waite KA, Eng C. Nuclear localization of PTEN is regulated by Ca(2+) through a tyrosil phosphorylation-independent conformational modification in major vault protein. Cancer Res. 2006;66:11677–82.
144. Chu EC, Tarnawski AS. PTEN regulatory functions in tumor suppression and cell biology. Med Sci Monit. 2004;10:RA235–41.
145. Weng LP, Smith WM, Brown JL, Eng C. PTEN inhibits insulin-stimulated MEK/MAPK activation and cell growth by blocking IRS-1 phosphorylation and IRS-1/Grb-2/Sos complex formation in a breast cancer model. Hum Mol Genet. 2001;10:605–16.
146. Zhang S, Yu D. PI(3)king apart PTEN's role in cancer. Clin Cancer Res. 2010;16:4325–30.
147. Bonneau D, Longy M. Mutations of the human PTEN gene. Hum Mutat. 2000;16:109–22.
148. Orloff MS, Eng C. Genetic and phenotypic heterogeneity in the PTEN hamartoma tumour syndrome. Oncogene. 2008;27:5387–97.
149. Zbuk KM, Eng C. Cancer phenomics: RET and PTEN as illustrative models. Nat Rev Cancer. 2007;7:35–45.
150. Marsh DJ, Coulon V, Lunetta KL, Rocca-Serra P, Dahia PL, Zheng Z, Liaw D, Caron S, Duboue B, Lin AY, et al. Mutation spectrum and genotype-phenotype analyses in Cowden disease and Bannayan-Zonana syndrome, two hamartoma syndromes with germline PTEN mutation. Hum Mol Genet. 1998;7:507–15.
151. Zhou XP, Waite KA, Pilarski R, Hampel H, Fernandez MJ, Bos C, Dasouki M, Feldman GL, Greenberg LA, Ivanovich J, et al. Germline PTEN promoter mutations and deletions in Cowden/Bannayan-Riley-Ruvalcaba syndrome result in aberrant PTEN protein and dysregulation of the phosphoinositol-3-kinase/Akt pathway. Am J Hum Genet. 2003;73:404–11.

152. Loffeld A, McLellan NJ, Cole T, Payne SJ, Fricker D, Moss C. Epidermal naevus in Proteus syndrome showing loss of heterozygosity for an inherited PTEN mutation. Br J Dermatol. 2006;154:1194–8.
153. Smith JM, Kirk EP, Theodosopoulos G, Marshall GM, Walker J, Rogers M, Field M, Brereton JJ, Marsh DJ. Germline mutation of the tumour suppressor PTEN in Proteus syndrome. J Med Genet. 2002;39:937–40.
154. Zhou X, Hampel H, Thiele H, Gorlin RJ, Hennekam RC, Parisi M, Winter RM, Eng C. Association of germline mutation in the PTEN tumour suppressor gene and Proteus and Proteus-like syndromes. Lancet. 2001;358:210–1.
155. Thiffault I, Schwartz CE, Der Kaloustian V, Foulkes WD. Mutation analysis of the tumor suppressor PTEN and the glypican 3 (GPC3) gene in patients diagnosed with Proteus syndrome. Am J Med Genet A. 2004;130A:123–7.
156. Chibon F, Primois C, Bressieux JM, Lacombe D, Lok C, Mauriac L, Taieb A, Longy M. Contribution of PTEN large rearrangements in Cowden disease: a multiplex amplifiable probe hybridisation (MAPH) screening approach. J Med Genet. 2008;45:657–65.
157. Ni Y, Zbuk KM, Sadler T, Patocs A, Lobo G, Edelman E, Platzer P, Orloff MS, Waite KA, Eng C. Germline mutations and variants in the succinate dehydrogenase genes in Cowden and Cowden-like syndromes. Am J Hum Genet. 2008;83:261–8.
158. Nizialek EA, Mester JL, Dhiman VK, Smiraglia DJ, Eng C. KLLN epigenotype-phenotype associations in Cowden syndrome. Eur J Hum Genet. 2015;23:1538–43.
159. Zhou XP, Marsh DJ, Morrison CD, Chaudhury AR, Maxwell M, Reifenberger G, Eng C. Germline inactivation of PTEN and dysregulation of the phosphoinositol-3-kinase/Akt pathway cause human Lhermitte-Duclos disease in adults. Am J Hum Genet. 2003;73:1191–8.
160. Butler MG, Dasouki MJ, Zhou XP, Talebizadeh Z, Brown M, Takahashi TN, Miles JH, Wang CH, Stratton R, Pilarski R, et al. Subset of individuals with autism spectrum disorders and extreme macrocephaly associated with germline PTEN tumour suppressor gene mutations. J Med Genet. 2005;42:318–21.
161. Herman GE, Butter E, Enrile B, Pastore M, Prior TW, Sommer A. Increasing knowledge of PTEN germline mutations: two additional patients with autism and macrocephaly. Am J Med Genet A. 2007;143:589–93.
162. Herman GE, Henninger N, Ratliff-Schaub K, Pastore M, Fitzgerald S, McBride KL. Genetic testing in autism: how much is enough? Genet Med. 2007;9:268–74.
163. Orrico A, Galli L, Buoni S, Orsi A, Vonella G, Sorrentino V. Novel PTEN mutations in neurodevelopmental disorders and macrocephaly. Clin Genet. 2009;75:195–8.
164. Varga EA, Pastore M, Prior T, Herman GE, McBride KL. The prevalence of PTEN mutations in a clinical pediatric cohort with autism spectrum disorders, developmental delay, and macrocephaly. Genet Med. 2009;11:111–7.
165. Marsh DJ, Kum JB, Lunetta KL, Bennett MJ, Gorlin RJ, Ahmed SF, Bodurtha J, Crowe C, Curtis MA, Dasouki M, et al. PTEN mutation spectrum and genotype-phenotype correlations in Bannayan-Riley-Ruvalcaba syndrome suggest a single entity with Cowden syndrome. Hum Mol Genet. 1999;8:1461–72.
166. Kim S, Misra A. SNP genotyping: technologies and biomedical applications. Annu Rev Biomed Eng. 2007;9:289–320.
167. Morozova O, Marra MA. Applications of next-generation sequencing technologies in functional genomics. Genomics. 2008;92:255–64.

Chapter 5
Clinical Management and Treatment of Vascular Tumors

Kristin E. Holland and Beth A. Drolet

Infantile Hemangioma

Infantile hemangiomas (IHs), also known as hemangiomas of infancy, are the most common soft tissue tumor of childhood. Despite their frequency, much remains to be learned about the pathogenesis, and management is often based on anecdote rather than evidence-based data. While most IHs are uncomplicated and do not require intervention, they can be a significant source of parental distress, cosmetic disfigurement, and morbidity. The wide spectrum of disease both in the morphology of these lesions and more importantly in their behavior has made it difficult to predict need for treatment and has made it challenging to establish a standardized approach to management.

The clinical heterogeneity and unpredictable and variable course of IH complicate management decisions and have contributed to the lack of an evidenced-based standard of care. There are few prospective studies looking at safety and efficacy of therapies for IH, and no Food and Drug Administration (FDA)-approved agents for IH exist. As a result, selection of therapeutic modalities is based on anecdote and small case series. Physicians caring for an infant with IH must first determine whether treatment is indicated. Although most hemangiomas are self-limited, up to 38 % of hemangiomas referred to tertiary care specialists require systemic treatment due to complications such as ulceration, bleeding, risk for

K.E. Holland, MD (✉)
Pediatric Dermatology – Administrative Research Offices, Medical College of Wisconsin,
8701 Watertown Plank Road, TBRC, 2nd Fl, Suite C2010, 53226 Milwaukee, WI, USA
e-mail: kholland@mcw.edu

B.A. Drolet, MD
Dermatology Department, Division of Pediatric Dermatology, Medical College of Wisconsin,
Milwaukee, WI, USA

© Springer Science+Business Media New York 2016
P.E. North, T. Sander (eds.), *Vascular Tumors and Developmental Malformations*,
Molecular and Translational Medicine, DOI 10.1007/978-1-4939-3240-5_5

Table 5.1 Factors to consider in estimating potential need for treatment

Therapeutic consideration	Intervention more likely
Location at risk for complication, functional impairment, cosmetic disfigurement	See Table 5.2
Presence of ulceration	Symptomatic from pain, bleeding
Morphology of IH	Large, segmental Exophytic, sessile, or pedunculated lesions
Growth pattern	Rapid or prolonged
Age	Younger age = higher potential for growth School-age child with incomplete resolution or presence of residual IH

From Holland and Drolet [59]. Reprinted with permission from Elsevier Limited

Table 5.2 High-risk locations

Location	Associated risk
Periorbital and retrobulbar	Visual axis occlusion, astigmatism, amblyopia
Nasal tip, ear, large facial	Cosmetic disfigurement, scarring
Perioral, lip	Ulceration, feeding difficulties, cosmetic disfigurement
Perineal, axilla, neck	Ulceration
"Beard" distribution, central neck	Airway hemangioma
Liver, large	High-output heart failure
Multifocal or multiple	Visceral involvement (liver, gastrointestinal tract most common)
Midline lumbosacral	Tethered spinal cord, intraspinal hemangioma, intraspinal lipoma, genitourinary anomalies

From Holland and Drolet [59]. Reprinted with permission from Elsevier Limited

permanent disfigurement, obstruction of vision, airway obstruction, or high-output cardiac failure [1]. A number of factors outlined in Table 5.1 must be considered by physicians managing patients with IH.

Ulceration

Ulceration is the most common complication (16 %) and can be a significant source of pain, infection, bleeding, and permanent scarring [1]. Associated pain can interfere with sleep as well as feeding. Locations at high risk for ulceration and the associated frequency of this complication include anogenital (50 %), lower lip (30 %), and neck (25 %) [2]. Infantile hemangiomas which are larger in size or of the "segmental" subtype are more likely to develop ulceration. Of the clinical subtypes (i.e., superficial, mixed, and deep), the mixed subtype (having both superficial and deep components) has most frequently been associated with ulceration and is another independent risk factor [2, 3]. The cause of ulceration is not well understood, but maceration and friction are likely contributing factors given the higher frequency in locations prone to this. While ulceration can be complicated by bleeding, clinically significant bleeding (i.e., requiring hospitalization/transfusion) is rare [2].

Initial therapy for most ulcerated hemangiomas, a common indication for treatment, is local wound care. Gentle debridement of crust overlying the ulceration can be achieved with wet compresses with dilute hydrogen peroxide soaks or astringent solutions of aluminum acetate (i.e. Domeboro solution (Bayer HealthCare, Morristown, NJ)). In the diaper area, barrier creams containing zinc oxide or petrolatum play an important role in protecting the skin from maceration and irritation from urine and stool, which may inhibit healing. Nonadherent dressings such as petrolatum gauze or extrathin hydrocolloid dressings may act as an additional barrier to outside pathogens or irritants and promote healing. As secondary infection can develop in ulcerated IH, cultures should be obtained in nonhealing lesions recognizing that colonization is not uncommon and topical antibiotics (i.e. polymyxin-bacitracin, mupirocin, metronidazole) should be employed when indicated. Oral antibiotics may be necessary in patients nonresponsive to topical measures.

In ulcerations recalcitrant to initial topical measures outlined above, topical application of becaplermin gel, a recombinant human platelet-derived growth factor, has been shown in a small case series to be effective at speeding healing [4]. More recently, a boxed warning was placed on this medication about the possible increased risk of mortality secondary to malignancy in some adult patients. As a result, its role is generally reserved as a second- or third-line agent for patients who have failed other treatment modalities.

The pulsed dye laser may be helpful in healing ulcerated hemangiomas and is discussed later in the text in the section in which laser is discussed. Systemic medication is often needed to slow the proliferation of the hemangiomas and heal the ulceration. Ulceration in the midline face and of cartilage (nose, ears) is often very difficult to treat and even with aggressive topical and systemic therapy ulceration may persist.

Topical Therapy

Corticosteroids

Both topical and intralesional corticosteroids have a role in the management of IH and are discussed later in the section in which corticosteroids are discussed.

Imiquimod

Topical imiquimod (5 %), an immune response modifier, has been reported to result in improvement in infantile hemangiomas in several case reports and small uncontrolled case series [5–10]. Its antiangiogenic activity is thought to occur as the result of a combination of activation of the innate immune system through Toll-like receptor-7 (TLR-7) to induce interferon alpha (IFN-α), tumor necrosis factor alpha (TNFα), interferon gamma, and tissue inhibitor of matrix metalloproteinase as well as through intrinsic proapoptotic activity [7, 9]. Successful treatment of IH with systemic IFN-α is associated with a decrease of vascular endothelial growth factor (VEGF) and basic fibroblast growth factor (bFGF) within the IH and in blood [9]. In a Phase II, open-label study of topical imiquimod in the treatment of nonulcerated superficial and mixed IH, serum levels of IFN-α were mostly undetectable, and all were well below peak levels described with systemic IFN-α [6, 9]. In addition, no correlation was observed between clinical response to topical imiquimod and VEGF and bFGF levels in urine or blood. While shrinkage and flattening of IH has been observed with the use of imiquimod cream [6], no significant changes were observed in lesion area, volume, depth, or elevation in the Phase II, open-label study. A greater response was seen in superficial IH compared to mixed lesions, mainly in regard to color [7, 9]. Reported treatment regimens often start with application of imiquimod 3 times/week overnight, increasing to 5–7 times/week after 4 weeks if no response is seen [7, 9]. Local side effects are common which include edema, erythema, scaliness, and crusting at the site of treatment [6, 7, 9, 10]. Such an inflammatory response seems to correlate with response of the IH given the absence of redness and crusting in recalcitrant lesions [10]. Residual hypopigmented scars have been described in a patient with severe crusting [9]. The local side effects and poor therapeutic response have made this treatment modality obsolete.

Timolol

In 2008, systemic propranolol was first reported to result in improvement in IH, and it is currently widely used [11]. The use of systemic propranolol in the management of IH is discussed in detail later in this chapter. More recently, twice daily application of a topical β-blocker, timolol maleate 0.5 % ophthalmic solution (two drops twice daily) and gel, has been reported to result in improvement in size, thickness, and color of superficial IH in a single case report and in a small pilot study [12, 13]. Future studies will better establish the safety and efficacy of this medication and define its role in the management of IH.

Systemic Therapy

Corticosteroids

Oral corticosteroids at a dose of 2–5 mg/kg/day (typically 2–3 mg/kg/day) have historically been the mainstay of therapy. Patients are typically maintained on this dose for 1–3 months and then slowly tapered over several months [14]. The duration of treatment and approach to tapering corticosteroids is variable, as it is dependent on the treatment response, age of the child, inherent growth characteristics of the IH, and complications of therapy. For example, younger infants tend to be treated longer (months) given their greater potential for IH growth, whereas older infants whose IH may be nearing the end of its proliferative phase would be less likely to need prolonged therapy. Response to treatment is variable. A quantitative systematic review of the literature identified 10 case series representing 184 patients in which systemic corticosteroids were used in the management of IH; mean response rate was 84 % (range 60–100 %) and a dose–response relationship was confirmed with higher response rates (as defined by cessation of growth or reduction in size coincident with initiation of treatment) noted in patients treated with higher dose prednisone/prednisolone (>3 mg/kg/day compared to 0–2 mg/kg/day) [15]. A more recent randomized, controlled trial evaluated daily oral prednisolone (2 mg/kg/day) compared to monthly intravenous pulses of methylprednisolone (30 mg/kg/day for 3 consecutive days each month) for 3 months [14]. Greater improvement was noted in the oral prednisolone group compared to the intravenous group at 3 months and 1 year (median visual analog score of 70 vs 12 and 50 vs −1.5, respectively). Adverse effects are common and include irritability, gastrointestinal upset, sleep disturbance, cushingoid facies, adrenal suppression, immunosuppression, hypertension, bone demineralization, cardiomyopathy, and growth retardation [16]. Catch-up growth occurs in the majority of children once the corticosteroids are discontinued [17, 18]. A prospective study of 16 infants evaluating the immunosuppressive effects of corticosteroids demonstrated that both lymphocyte cell numbers and function are affected [19]. As the levels of tetanus and diphtheria antibodies were not found to be protective in 11 and 3 of the patients, respectively, it has been recommended that patients who receive oral corticosteroids during the immunization period have these checked and additional immunizations provided if titers are not protective. In addition, prophylaxis with a combination of trimethoprim and sulfamethoxazole should be considered in infants to protect against *Pneumocystis* pneumonia (PCP) as there are reports of PCP in this setting [20].

Intralesional and topical corticosteroids have also been reported to decrease the size or slow growth of IH and may be an alternative to systemic therapy in lower-risk lesions. This is most effective for localized and superficial cutaneous hemangiomas. The efficacy of topical corticosteroids is limited by the depth of its penetration compared to the depth of hemangioma involvement. There have been small case series and a larger (34 patients) retrospective study in which ultrapotent topical corticosteroids (clobetasol propionate, halobetasol propionate, and augmented betamethasone dipropionate) were used to treat infantile hemangiomas [21–23]. In these reports, lightening of the superficial component was seen most commonly with cessation of growth or shrinkage being reported less frequently. Dosing regimens varied from once to twice daily application and durations ranging from continuous therapy with close monitoring to 2–4 week cycles of active treatment separated by 1 week without treatment. No evidence of hypothalamic-pituitary-adrenal axis suppression was found, but this was not routinely evaluated [22, 23]. Response to intralesional triamcinolone is not surprisingly faster, but has a higher side effect profile. Central retinal artery occlusion and blindness, believed to be the result of pressure exceeding systolic pressure during injection, have been reported in the treatment of periocular hemangiomas, limiting its use in this location [16]. Other complications related to intralesional corticosteroids include skin atrophy and necrosis, calcification, and, rarely, adrenal suppression (dose dependent). Doses of intralesional triamcinolone should not exceed 3–5 mg/kg per treatment [16]. Rebound growth with both topical and intralesional treatment may be seen, and repeated injections or courses of topical therapy are often necessary to maintain response.

Propranolol

Propranolol has recently been utilized in the treatment of infantile hemangiomas after growth arrest of an infant's hemangioma was incidentally noted when propranolol was started for obstructive hypertrophic myocardiopathy [11]. Improvement in color, softening, growth arrest, and even regression of IH have been observed with administration of propranolol [11, 24]. Since the initial report, the use of propranolol for IH has soared, as it is perceived to have a lower side effect profile than other systemic therapies used for treating IH. Its mechanism of action in the treatment of IH is unknown, but there are a number of proposed effects including vasoconstriction, decreased expression of vascular endothelial growth factor (VEGF) and basic fibroblast growth factor (bFGF), and apoptosis of capillary endothelial cells [13]. In addition to a number of case reports in the literature, two retrospective studies (including a total of 62 patients) have reported the successful use of propranolol in the management of IH with cessation of growth, lightening of color, softening, and healing of superficial ulcers [25, 26]. Doses of 1–3 mg/kg/day divided bid or tid have typically been used, but clearly outlined and safe protocols for initiation and monitoring do not exist resulting in a wide range in recommendations. The most common serious side effects of propranolol include bradycardia and hypotension. Other side effects include bronchospasm (particularly in patients with reactive airway disease), congestive heart failure, depression, nausea, vomiting, abdominal cramping, sleep disturbance, and night terrors. Hypoglycemia, particularly after overnight fast, may be observed [27]. The most common side effect reported in one retrospective study was somnolence [25], a potential sign of hypoglycemia; glucose monitoring was not reported to be part of the routine evaluation in this study.

There are theoretical considerations specific to using oral propranolol for the treatment of IH (Table 5.3). Regarding hypoglycemia, most patients will be less than 1 year of age and have limited glycogen stores and a relative inability to communicate, recognize, or treat symptoms. Furthermore, low birth weight, an important risk factor for the development of IH, also confers a greater risk of hypoglycemia. Oral corticosteroids are used frequently for the treatment of infantile hemangiomas; during treatment, there may be some protective effect as steroids inhibit insulin action. However, after prolonged steroid use, there may be

Table 5.3 Patients with theoretical increased risk of adverse effects from propranolol for IH

Population	Side effect	Reason for concern
<1 year of age *Particularly LBW infants	Hypoglycemia	Limited glycogen stores Inability to communicate symptoms
Patients previously treated with systemic steroids	Hypoglycemia	Muted counter-regulatory cortisol response secondary to adrenal suppression
PHACE syndrome patients with cerebrovascular anomalies	Hypoperfusion of brain	Narrowed, stenotic vessels may require higher blood pressure for perfusion; propranolol associated with decreased cerebral blood flow
PHACE syndrome patients with aortic arch obstruction	Systemic hypoperfusion	Aortic obstruction may require higher blood pressure to maintain perfusion to segments distal to the obstruction
Hemangioma-related high-output cardiac failure (i.e., large liver hemangioma)	Decompensation of heart failure	Decreased heart rate/contractility limits cardiac response to high output demands

From Holland and Drolet [59]. Reprinted with permission from Elsevier Limited

LBW low birth weight

residual adrenal suppression and subsequent loss of the counter-regulatory corti-sol response, thus increasing risk of hypoglycemia. In patients with PHACE syn-drome and cerebrovascular or aortic arch anomalies, lower blood pressure may decrease blood flow through stenotic or dysplastic vessels resulting in hypoperfu-sion of the brain (when cerebrovascular vessels are involved) or the lower body (when aortic coarctation is present). Finally, in patients with high-output cardiac failure secondary to a large liver hemangioma, the use of propranolol could result in decompensation secondary to drug-induced suppression of heart rate/contractil-ity. Until the safety of propranolol in these patients can be established and these theoretic concerns allayed, caution should be exercised when prescribing propranolol.

Vincristine

Vincristine is a vinca alkaloid which disrupts the mitotic spindle and interferes with mitosis resulting in apoptosis. It has also shown efficacy as an antiangiogenic agent [28]. It has been reported to be effective in the treatment of IH and has historically been reserved for those IH resistant to corticosteroids or in patients intolerant of corticosteroids. While there are several case reports indicating improvement in "hemangiomas" with vincristine, these often represent other vascular tumors, and knowledge about its use for infantile hemangioma is limited. Single weekly doses of 1–1.5 mg/m^2 resulted in improvement of all nine patients reported by Enjolras and a patient reported by Fawcett [29, 30]. Constipation is the most common side effect, but neuromyopathy, most commonly presenting as foot drop, is a potentially serious side effect. Administration of vincristine requires placement of a central line; therefore, risks associated with this must be considered as well.

Interferon

Recombinant interferon alpha (IFN-α), an inhibitor of angiogenesis, administered as a subcutaneous injection of 3 million units per square meter per day, has also been used successfully for the treatment of IH [16]. Side effects include flu-like symptoms of fever, irritability, and malaise. Less commonly, transient neutropenia and liver enzyme abnormalities may be develop. Spastic diplegia, irreversible in some cases, has also been a reported side effect. The development of spastic diplegia has been observed more frequently in infants treated at an earlier age, the time at which there is often greatest need for treatment. Consequently, its use is not recommended in infants less than 9 months of age.

Laser

The pulsed dye laser (PDL) has been successfully used for vascular birthmarks, namely, capillary malformations or "port-wine stains" for years, and its efficacy in this setting is well established. Its use in the treatment of proliferating IH remains controversial as adverse outcomes including ulceration and scarring have been described [31]. In addition, the use of PDL for intact IH is limited by the depth of the laser's penetration (1 mm). A controlled trial in which 121 infants with IH were randomized to either treatment with the pulsed dye laser or observation showed no significant difference in clearance of the IH at 1 year [32]. Patients in the treatment group did demonstrate decreased redness compared to the untreated group, but at the expense of having a higher incidence of atrophy and hypopigmentation. There are a number of reports and two prospective studies describing its benefit in the treatment of ulcerated hemangiomas both in terms of speeding reepithelialization and decreasing pain [33, 34]. The mechanism for this is not well understood. Greatest consensus surrounding the use of the PDL for IH is in the treatment of residual telangiectases after involution, for which the PDL is most effective.

Surgery

Surgical excision may be an option for function- or life-threatening hemangiomas when medical therapy fails or is not tolerated, but more commonly its role is for removal of residual fibrofatty tissue or correction of scarring after involution.

Surgical correction may be pursued at an earlier age if it is clear that the child will ultimately need a procedure for the residual effects. Surgical excision may also be considered as a first-line therapy in select sites (scalp, neck, diaper area, and trunk) given the lower risk of surgical scar.

Kaposiform Hemangioendothelioma and Tufted Angioma With and Without Kasabach-Merritt Phenomenon

Kasabach-Merritt phenomenon (KMP) is a life-threatening, consumptive coagulopathy associated with an underlying vascular tumor [35]. Kasabach and Merritt first described this consumptive coagulopathy in a 2-month-old male with a giant "capillary hemangioma and purpura" [35]. Major developments in the study of vascular anomalies have led to a much clearer understanding of this phenomenon and the associated coagulopathy. Infantile hemangiomas (IH) are now recognized to be a unique vascular tumor which can be distinguished histologically from other vascular tumors and malformations by the presence of immunohistochemical staining with Glut-1 and other markers [36, 37]. Recent studies demonstrate the association of KMP with the vascular tumors, kaposiform hemangioendothelioma (KHE) and tufted angioma (TA), not infantile hemangioma [38–40].

KMP is characterized by severe thrombocytopenia, microangiopathic anemia, hypofibrinogenemia, and elevated fibrin split products (FSP) in the presence of an enlarging vascular tumor [41]. The coagulopathy is likely related to the sequestration of platelets and clotting factors within the vascular lesion resulting in systemic disseminated intravascular coagulation and a high propensity for patients to clot and bleed [42].

Clinical Presentation

KMP typically has its onset early in infancy with a median age of onset of 5 weeks [43]. In approximately 50 % of cases, KMP was associated with a vascular tumor diagnosed at birth with 90 % of published cases diagnosed before 1 year of age [36–38, 43, 44]. Boys and girls were equally affected. KMP was most often associated with a large solitary tumor commonly involving extremities, axilla, groin, or lateral face and neck. Most of these tumors are firm and have a nodular or even pebble-like texture. The skin over the tumors is deep red to purple in color often with subtle hypertrichosis. Occasionally, hyperhidrosis is noted over the surface of the tumor. If thrombocytopenia is severe, the surface of the tumor and the surrounding skin are ecchymotic. They may be localized to the skin, but often involve subcutaneous and deep structures. Widespread cutaneous petechiae may be seen in patients with platelet counts less than 10,000. Signs and symptoms of bleeding are seen in over 50 % of children with KMP at presentation in one report [44]. Patients with retroperitoneal or visceral lesions presented with abdominal distention, signs of organ dysfunction, and/or high-output heart failure often without cutaneous signs [36, 38, 44]. Patients with KMP have anemia, profound thrombocytopenia, and hypofibrinogenemia with elevated fibrin split products or D-dimers suggestive of a very active consumptive coagulopathy. Platelet counts at the time of diagnosis ranged from 6000 to 98,000 with fibrinogen levels less than 100 mg/dL while D-dimers were always >1 [36, 38, 44].

MRI is the best modality to assess vascular tumors associated with KMP. These tumors are diffusely enhancing masses isointense to muscle on T1 and hyperintense on T2-weighted sequences [36]. They involve multiple tissue planes and have poorly defined margins with finger-like extensions. Cutaneous thickening and fat stranding are common features [36]. Superficial draining vessels are often dilated, but vessels in the tumor are small and infrequent.

Vascular Pathology Associated with KMP

Several studies in the 1990s challenged the long held belief that KMP was a complication of infantile hemangiomas and definitively established the association of KMP with kaposiform hemangioendothelioma (KHE) and tufted angioma (TA) [36, 45, 46]. Of the 40 biopsy samples from 52 patients in these studies, 35 were diagnosed with KHE while 5 were called TA. Since then, biopsies of most lesions associated with KMP have shared the same histopathologic features [38, 42, 44, 47]. Not all patients diagnosed with TA or KHE have an associated consumptive coagulopathy arguing that other features such as age of the patient, tumor size, or location may be important risk factors for KMP. In our experience, KHE or TA localized to the skin and soft tissue is less likely to be associated with KMP.

Treatment

Pharmacologic intervention is not always necessary for TA/KHE. The natural history of these vascular tumors is highly variable; smaller tumors localized to the skin only may grow very slowly or even spontaneously involute. Treatment is indicated if there is pain, rapid growth, local invasion causing functional impairment, or if KMP is present. KMP is associated with significant morbidity and mortality; infants with KMP can die from hemorrhage or invasion/compression of vital structures by the tumor. Mortality from KMP has ranged between 10 % and 30 % in most series [36–38, 42, 44, 45, 48]. The management of KMP should include supportive care to maintain hemostasis and curative therapy directed at the treatment of the underlying tumor. Despite marked thrombocytopenia at presentation, platelet transfusions should be reserved for active bleeding. Infused platelets have a very short circulatory time and have been noted to rapidly increase the size of the tumor and even exacerbate KMP in some cases presumably through increased platelet trapping within the lesion [49–51]. Successful treatment of the underlying vascular tumor is critical to the correction of KMP and to the overall survival of the patient. A number of therapies have been reported for KHE/TA, but none have been uniformly effective. Although surgical removal of the tumor has been associated with immediate normalization of hemostasis and hematologic abnormalities [52], it is rarely feasible due to the large size and infiltrative nature of KHE/TA associated with KMP. Tumor embolization has been used with some success in combination with medical and surgical therapies [44]. Medical therapies have included cortico-steroids, interferon alpha (IFN-α), vincristine, as well as other chemotherapy agents used alone and in combination with varying results [53–55]. First-line therapy with corticosteroids at doses ranging from 2 to 30 mg/kg/day resulted in improved hematological parameters in 10–30 % of patients within days of starting therapy with little effect on tumor size [36]. IFN-α alone or in combination with steroids resulted in resolution of coagulopathy and tumor regression in approximately 40 % of patients [36]. However, the significant risk of irreversible neurotoxicity (spastic diplegia) in young infants treated with IFN-α has tempered its use [56]. Vincristine is emerging as a safe and effective treatment for KMP. All 15 patients in one series treated with vincristine as front-line therapy either alone or in combination with other agents responded with improved coagulation and hematologic parameters, while 13 showed significant reductions in tumor size [57].

Despite cure of KMP, most patients remain with a large residual tumor after medical or interventional radiology therapies [45]. These quiescent tumors can progress, often resulting in pain, functional impairment, and in rare instances a late relapse of KMP [45, 58]. Significant late effects in this population highlight the need for long-term follow-up and a better understanding of the unique biology of KHE/TA to facilitate the development of new (targeted) therapies resulting in more complete resolution of the underlying malignancy.

References

1. Haggstrom AN, Drolet BA, Baselga E, et al. Prospective study of infantile hemangiomas: clinical characteristics predicting complications and treatment. Pediatrics. 2006;118(3):882–7.
2. Chamlin SL, Haggstrom AN, Drolet BA, et al. Multicenter prospective study of ulcerated hemangiomas. J Pediatr. 2007;151(6):684. e-689.
3. Shin HT, Orlow SJ, Chang MW. Ulcerated haemangioma of infancy: a retrospective review of 47 patients. Br J Dermatol. 2007;156(5):1050–2.
4. Metz BJ, Rubenstein MC, Levy ML, Metry DW. Response of ulcerated perineal hemangiomas of infancy to becaplermin gel, a recombinant human platelet-derived growth factor. Arch Dermatol. 2004;140(7):867–70.
5. Barry RB, Hughes BR, Cook LJ. Involution of infantile haemangiomas after imiquimod 5% cream. Clin Exp Dermatol. 2008;33(4):446–9.
6. Hazen PG, Carney JF, Engstrom CW, Turgeon KL, Reep MD, Tanphaichitr A. Proliferating hemangioma of infancy: successful treatment with topical 5% imiquimod cream. Pediatr Dermatol. 2005;22(3):254–6.

7. Ho NT, Lansang P, Pope E. Topical imiquimod in the treatment of infantile hemangiomas: a retrospective study. J Am Acad Dermatol. 2007;56(1):63–8.
8. Martinez MI, Sanchez-Carpintero I, North PE, Mihm Jr MC. Infantile hemangioma: clinical resolution with 5% imiquimod cream. Arch Dermatol. 2002;138(7):881–4.
9. McCuaig CC, Dubois J, Powell J, et al. A phase II, open-label study of the efficacy and safety of imiquimod in the treatment of superficial and mixed infantile hemangioma. Pediatr Dermatol. 2009;26(2):203–12.
10. Welsh O, Olazaran Z, Gomez M, Salas J, Berman B. Treatment of infantile hemangiomas with short-term application of imiquimod 5% cream. J Am Acad Dermatol. 2004;51(4):639–42.
11. Leaute-Labreze C, Dumas de la Roque E, Hubiche T, Boralevi F, Thambo JB, Taieb A. Propranolol for severe hemangiomas of infancy. N Engl J Med. 2008;358(24):2649–51.
12. Guo S, Ni N. Topical treatment for capillary hemangioma of the eyelid using beta-blocker solution. Arch Ophthalmol. 2010;128(2):255–6.
13. Pope E, Chakkittakandiyil A. Topical timolol gel for infantile hemangiomas: a pilot study. Arch Dermatol. 2010;146(5):564–5.
14. Pope E, Krafchik BR, Macarthur C, et al. Oral versus high-dose pulse corticosteroids for problematic infantile hemangiomas: a randomized, controlled trial. Pediatrics. 2007;119(6):e1239–47.
15. Bennett ML, Fleischer Jr AB, Chamlin SL, Frieden IJ. Oral corticosteroid use is effective for cutaneous hemangiomas: an evidence-based evaluation. Arch Dermatol. 2001;137(9):1208–13.
16. Barrio VR, Drolet BA. Treatment of hemangiomas of infancy. Dermatol Ther. 2005; 18(2):151–9.
17. Boon LM, MacDonald DM, Mulliken JB. Complications of systemic corticosteroid therapy for problematic hemangioma. Plast Reconstr Surg. 1999;104(6):1616–23.
18. Lomenick JP, Backeljauw PF, Lucky AW. Growth, bone mineral accretion, and adrenal function in glucocorticoid-treated infants with hemangiomas – a retrospective study. Pediatr Dermatol. 2006;23(2):169–74.
19. Kelly ME, Juern AM, Grossman WJ, Schauer DW, Drolet BA. Immunosuppressive effects in infants treated with corticosteroids for infantile hemangiomas. Arch Dermatol. 2010;146(7):767–74.
20. Maronn ML, Corden T, Drolet BA. Pneumocystis carinii pneumonia in infant treated with oral steroids for hemangioma. Arch Dermatol. 2007;143(9):1224–5.
21. Elsas FJ, Lewis AR. Topical treatment of periocular capillary hemangioma. J Pediatr Ophthalmol Strabismus. 1994;31(3):153–6.
22. Cruz OA, Zarnegar SR, Myers SE. Treatment of periocular capillary hemangioma with topical clobetasol propionate. Ophthalmology. 1995;102(12):2012–5.
23. Garzon MC, Lucky AW, Hawrot A, Frieden IJ. Ultrapotent topical corticosteroid treatment of hemangiomas of infancy. J Am Acad Dermatol. 2005;52(2):281–6.
24. Sans V, Dumas de la Roque E, Berge J, et al. Propranolol for severe infantile hemangiomas: follow-up report. Pediatrics. 2009;124(3):e423–31.
25. Buckmiller LM, Munson PD, Dyamenahalli U, Dai Y, Richter GT. Propranolol for infantile hemangiomas: early experience at a tertiary vascular anomalies center. Laryngoscope. 2010;120(4):676–81.
26. Manunza F, Syed S, Laguda B, et al. Propranolol for complicated infantile haemangiomas: a case series of 30 infants. Br J Dermatol. 2010;162(2):466–8.
27. Holland KE, Frieden IJ, Frommelt PC, Mancini AJ, Wyatt D, Drolet BA. Hypoglycemia in children taking propranolol for the treatment of infantile hemangioma. Arch Dermatol. 2010;146(7):775–8.
28. Perez-Valle S, Peinador M, Herraiz P, Saenz P, Montoliu G, Vento M. Vincristine, an efficacious alternative for diffuse neonatal haemangiomatosis. Acta Paediatr. 2010;99(2):311–5.
29. Enjolras O, Breviere GM, Roger G, et al. Vincristine treatment for function- and life-threatening infantile hemangioma. Arch Pediatr. 2004;11:99–107.
30. Fawcett SL, Grant I, Hall PN, Kelsall AW, Nicholson JC. Vincristine as a treatment for a large haemangioma threatening vital functions. Br J Plast Surg. 2004;57(2):168–71.

31. Witman PM, Wagner AM, Scherer K, Waner M, Frieden IJ. Complications following pulsed dye laser treatment of superficial hemangiomas. Lasers Surg Med. 2006;38(2):116–23.
32. Batta K, Goodyear HM, Moss C, Williams HC, Hiller L, Waters R. Randomised controlled study of early pulsed dye laser treatment of uncomplicated childhood haemangiomas: results of a 1-year analysis. Lancet. 2002;360(9332):521–7.
33. David LR, Malek MM, Argenta LC. Efficacy of pulse dye laser therapy for the treatment of ulcerated haemangiomas: a review of 78 patients. Br J Plast Surg. 2003;56(4):317–27.
34. Morelli JG, Tan OT, Yohn JJ, Weston WL. Treatment of ulcerated hemangiomas infancy. Arch Pediatr Adolesc Med. 1994;148(10):1104–5.
35. Kasabach HH, Merritt KK. Capillary hemangioma with extensive purpura. Am J Dis Child. 1940;59:1063–79.
36. North PE, Waner M, Mizeracki A, Mihm Jr MC. GLUT1: a newly discovered immunohisto-chemical marker for juvenile hemangiomas. Hum Pathol. 2000;31(1):11–22.
37. North PE, Waner M, Mizeracki A, et al. A unique microvascular phenotype shared by juvenile hemangiomas and human placenta. Arch Dermatol. 2001;137(5):559–70.
38. Sarkar M, Mulliken JB, Kozakewich HP, Robertson RL, Burrows PE. Thrombocytopenic coagulopathy (Kasabach-Merritt phenomenon) is associated with kaposiform hemangio-endothelioma and not with common infantile hemangioma. Plast Reconstr Surg. 1997; 100(6):1377–86.
39. Enjolras O, Wassef M, Mazoyer E, et al. Infants with Kasabach-Merritt syndrome do not have "true" hemangiomas. J Pediatr. 1997;130(4):631–40.
40. Alvarez-Mendoza A, Lourdes TS, Ridaura-Sanz C, Ruiz-Maldonado R. Histopathology of vascular lesions found in Kasabach-Merritt syndrome: review based on 13 cases. Pediatr Dev Pathol. 2000;3(6):556–60.
41. Hall GW. Kasabach-Merritt syndrome: pathogenesis and management. Br J Haematol. 2001;112(4):851–62.
42. Lyons LL, North PE, Mac-Moune Lai F, Stoler MH, Folpe AL, Weiss SW. Kaposiform heman-gioendothelioma: a study of 33 cases emphasizing its pathologic, immunophenotypic, and biologic uniqueness from juvenile hemangioma. Am J Surg Pathol. 2004;28(5):559–68.
43. Shim WK. Hemangiomas of infancy complicated by thrombocytopenia. Am J Surg. 1968;116(6):896–906.
44. Ryan C, Price V, John P, et al. Kasabach-Merritt phenomenon: a single centre experience. Eur J Haematol. 2010;84(2):97–104.
45. Enjolras O, Mulliken JB, Wassef M, et al. Residual lesions after kasabach-merritt phenomenon in 41 patients. J Am Acad Dermatol. 2000;42(2 Pt 1):225–35.
46. Zukerberg LR, Nickoloff BJ, Weiss SW. Kaposiform hemangioendothelioma of infancy and childhood. an aggressive neoplasm associated with Kasabach-Merritt syndrome and lymphan-giomatosis. Am J Surg Pathol. 1993;17(4):321–8.
47. Rodriguez V, Lee A, Witman PM, Anderson PA. Kasabach-Merritt phenomenon: case series and retrospective review of the mayo clinic experience. J Pediatr Hematol Oncol. 2009; 31(7):522–6.
48. Verheul HM, Panigrahy D, Flynn E, Pinedo HM, D'Amato RJ. Treatment of the Kasabach-Merritt syndrome with pegylated recombinant human megakaryocyte growth and development factor in mice: elevated platelet counts, prolonged survival, and tumor growth inhibition. Pediatr Res. 1999;46(5):562–5.
49. Phillips WG, Marsden JR. Kasabach-Merritt syndrome exacerbated by platelet transfusion. J R Soc Med. 1993;86(4):231–2.
50. Pampin C, Devillers A, Treguier C, et al. Intratumoral consumption of indium-111-labeled platelets in a child with splenic hemangioma and thrombocytopenia. J Pediatr Hematol Oncol. 2000;22(3):256–8.
51. Seo SK, Suh JC, Na GY, Kim IS, Sohn KR. Kasabach-Merritt syndrome: identification of platelet trapping in a tufted angioma by immunohistochemistry technique using monoclonal antibody to CD61. Pediatr Dermatol. 1999;16(5):392–4.

52. Beaubien ER, Ball NJ, Storwick GS. Kaposiform hemangioendothelioma: a locally aggressive vascular tumor. J Am Acad Dermatol. 1998;38(5 Pt 2):799–802.
53. Perez Payarols J, Pardo Masferrer J, Gomez Bellvert C. Treatment of life-threatening infantile hemangiomas with vincristine. N Engl J Med. 1995;333(1):69.
54. Hu B, Lachman R, Phillips J, Peng SK, Sieger L. Kasabach-Merritt syndrome-associated kaposiform hemangioendothelioma successfully treated with cyclophosphamide, vincristine, and actinomycin D. J Pediatr Hematol Oncol. 1998;20(6):567–9.
55. Vin-Christian K, McCalmont TH, Frieden IJ. Kaposiform hemangioendothelioma. An aggressive, locally invasive vascular tumor that can mimic hemangioma of infancy. Arch Dermatol. 1997;133(12):1573–8.
56. Barlow CF, Priebe CJ, Mulliken JB, et al. Spastic diplegia as a complication of interferon alfa-2a treatment of hemangiomas of infancy. J Pediatr. 1998;132(3 Pt 1):527–30.
57. Haisley-Royster C, Enjolras O, Frieden IJ, et al. Kasabach-Merritt phenomenon: a retrospective study of treatment with vincristine. J Pediatr Hematol Oncol. 2002;24(6): 459–62.
58. Ohtsuka T, Saegusa M, Yamakage A, Yamazaki S. Angioblastoma (nakagawa) with hyperhidrosis, and relapse after a 10-year interval. Br J Dermatol. 2000;143(1):223–4.
59. Holland KE, Drolet BA. Infantile hemangioma. Pediatr Clin. 2010;57(5):1069–83.

Index

© Springer Science+Business Media New York 2016
P.E. North, T. Sander (eds.), *Vascular Tumors and Developmental Malformations,
Molecular and Translational Medicine*, DOI 10.1007/978-1-4939-3240-5

145

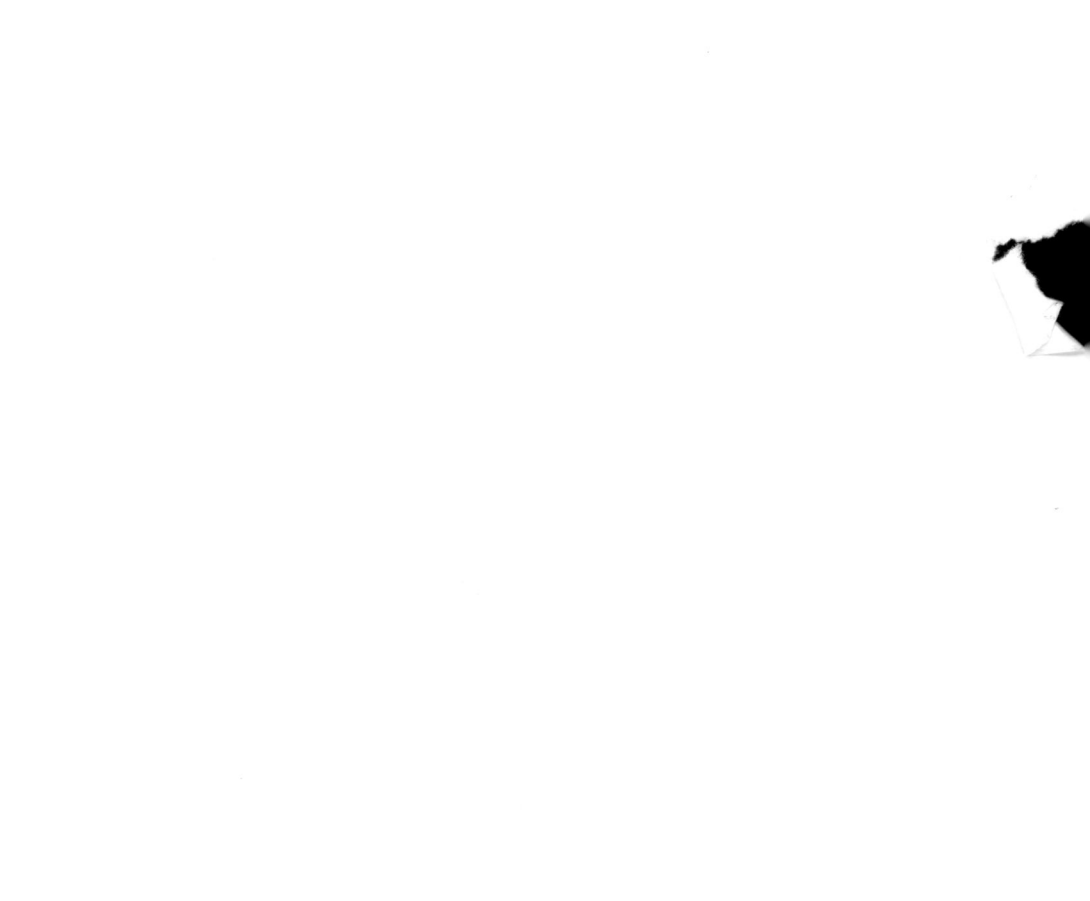